Your Journey to Aging Well

Thank you for purchasing this book. My hope is that every reader will find ways to be in control of their health for a long and happy life journey.

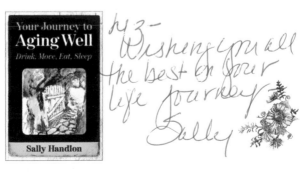

Your Journey to
Aging Well
Drink, Move, Eat, Sleep

Sally Handlon

*MZ —
Wishing you all
the best on your
life journey
Sally*

Your Journey to
Aging Well
Drink, Move, Eat, Sleep

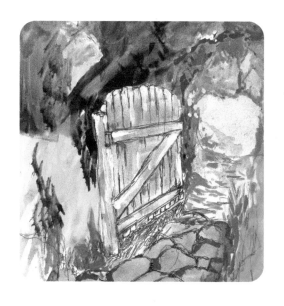

Sally Handlon

© 2020 by Sally Handlon

All rights reserved. No part of this publication may be reproduced or transmitted in any form or by any means, electronic or mechanical, including photocopying, recording, or any other information storage and retrieval system, without the written permission of the publisher.

This book is intended as a reference volume only, not as a medical manual. The information given here is designed to help you make informed decisions about your health. It is not intended as a substitute for any treatment that may have been prescribed by your doctor. If you suspect that you have a medical problem, we urge you to seek competent medical help.

Internet addresses given in this book were accurate at the time it went to press.

Printed in the United States of America

Published in Hellertown, PA

Edited by Jennifer Bright

Proofread by Skye Cruz

Cover and interior design by Christina Gaugler

Art by Robert L. Huetter

Library of Congress Control Number 2020901851

ISBN 978-1-7323016-0-3

2 4 6 8 10 9 7 5 3 1 paperback

I couldn't have navigated the path to writing this book without the help of several special people. I would like to dedicate this book to them.

My mother, Dorothy Abbott Manson,
who until her final days was an amazing lady

Justin Kelley, DC, chiropractor,
who introduced me to alternative medicine

David Winston, RH (AHG), world renowned herbalist,
whom I had the great fortune to study with

Joshua Rosenthal, founder and past director of the
Institute for Integrative Nutrition, whose work helped me
to understand the missing pieces to my learning

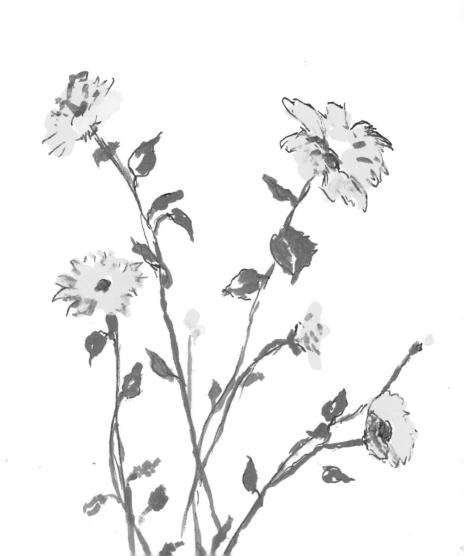

CONTENTS

A Note from the Author   9

Introduction   10

CHAPTER 1: Body Systems   15

CHAPTER 2: Drink   39

CHAPTER 3: Move   49

CHAPTER 4: Eat   61

CHAPTER 5: Sleep   77

Conclusion   87

References   88

Checklists   93

About the Author   99

About the Artist   101

A NOTE FROM THE AUTHOR

THIS BOOK IS A CULMINATION of more than 35 years of interest in health, environment, and wellness. Although I majored in physical education, then parks and recreation in college, I was young and didn't see these majors as a way to address wellness, nor did I really give thought to wellness. The real journey began with my subscription to *Prevention* magazine when I was in my early thirties. I continued to learn more about the body's capabilities through my work with a special alternative practitioner, Justin Kelley, DC.

This led to an interest in herbs as medicine and an introduction to herbalist David Winston, RH (AHG). Although I took three years of study with David's courses, I knew that I would always be a student herbalist. I realized that unless I devoted myself full time to this learning, I would remain a resource for family and friends only and never hang out a shingle.

Still, my journey wasn't over. It took me eight years to find the missing factor. It was discovering the connection between wellness, herbs, and nutrition that helped to forge my new path. My intent has always been to find a way to share the knowledge that I obtained, starting with the herbal training. While I was researching and writing this book, I realized that the seed for this book was planted many years ago, during my first year of herbal training. What a great find that was!

INTRODUCTION

"Listen to me and not to them."

—Gertrude Stein

OUR EARS WOULD FILL WITH ADVICE, if we listened to it. Advertisers, evangelists, publishers, educators, all clamoring to market their products, try to get us to conform to their notions of what we should be.

One of the dangers of a democratic society is confusing the individual and the mass—using statistical data to define persons instead of trends. "Trendiness" is a way of avoiding individuality. To choose for ourselves means taking responsibility for our choices, saying, "I do this because I want to."

Each of us has an interior voice that knows what we want. We know—even if the knowledge sometimes causes us pain—that we're unique individuals, with goals, programs, and behaviors distinct from others. Acknowledgment and enjoyment of our full humanity means owning our differences and listening to our own voices.

I am the expert on my own life. Today and every day, let me be wise enough to consult myself.[1]

Our bodies learn to adapt to our habits—whether those habits are good or bad. Unlike a car, where if you put in the wrong gas, it can immediately stop the function, the impact of bad health choices might not be felt for years.

However, there can be immediate consequences to bad habits. These include decreased energy, increased weight, and more frequent illnesses. Overtime, long-term bad health habits can lead to continuous inflammation, which may result in autoimmune type diseases.

What's amazing is that our bodies are fine-tuned "machines" designed to run efficiently and to heal themselves, given the proper nourishment—both food and lifestyle choices. When our choices are less than appropriate, we begin to erode our health and build inflammation.

If we take the time and desire to correct the fuel, most damage can be reversed. Two main contributors to this damage are eating food without the proper nutritional needs (eating chemicals instead of nutrients) and making lifestyle choices that increase daily stress—and sometimes lead to chronic stress.

First let's talk about the importance of making the most healthful food choices. If you can't pronounce the ingredients in a food, chances are that the body can't process them either. If your body can't process an ingredient, it's either excreted or stored in fat. David Winston, RH (AHG), herbalist and founder of the Center for Herbal Studies, is the person who made this statement really resonate with me: Just because something is "natural," it doesn't mean it is safe.

Second, consider the importance of making the most healthful lifestyle choices. Damage due to environmental toxins (especially an accumulation of pollutants), poor sleep, chronic stress, hyperglycemia, oxidative stress, copper toxicity (especially the brain mitochondria), heavy metals (such as nickel), and other factors lead to a loss of function.[2]

Everyone's needs are individual. They are based on your ancestry, family traditions, and body systems. No two people are exactly alike—not even identical twins. As Joshua Rosenthal, founder of the Institute for Integrative Nutrition often said, "One person's food can be another person's poison." He defined this as "bio individuality." That's why the choice of the foods that you eat and the lifestyle habits you choose (such as physical activity, relationships, spirituality, and career) should be unique to you. You may get guidance from other people or books; however, your implementation should be based on what works best for your body.

Today, Western medicine—through vaccines and antibiotics—has all but eliminated many of the infectious diseases that threatened our grandparents or great-grandparents at the turn off the twentieth century, including pneumonia, flu, and tuberculosis. Today, the top four diseases that we battle are all impacted by our lifestyle choices: heart disease, cancer, respiratory diseases, and stroke.

Another disease that's highly influenced by food and lifestyle choices is diabetes. And it's on the rise. The Centers for Disease Control and Prevention (CDC) predicts that one in three adults will have diabetes by 2050. Although the current rate for diabetes in adults is decreasing, the rate for youth is increasing. The next generation—our children and grandchildren—is anticipated to have a blighted future, facing a 35 percent increase in stroke, an 80 percent increase in heart disease, and a 90 percent increase in diabetes. These risks can be eliminated with changes in food and lifestyle.[3]

Plus, more than 80 autoimmune diseases occur as a result of your immune system attacking your body's own organs, tissues, and cells.

We're causing our own diseases. We need to shift that paradigm, and we can. Our bodies would like nothing better!

Unlike a new vehicle or appliance, your body didn't come with a warranty or guarantee. As choreographer and author Twyla Tharp said, "God gives you one gift; you get to be born. Thereafter you've got to take care of yourself."[4]

I can hear you objecting: But maybe I got bad genes! While it's true that genetics do play a role in health, your life choices have a greater impact. Isn't that empowering? You create your own health and wellness through the choices that you make each and every day.

But what about Father Time? True, you can't outrun him. But true biological aging is a surprisingly slow and graceful process, according to Henry S. Lodge, MD, coauthor of *Younger Next Year*.[5]

Hippocrates wrote, "Everyone has a doctor in him or her; we just have to help it in its work. The natural healing force within each of us is our greatest force in getting well."

This book is about helping each other get health! According to Mark Hyman, MD, just as chronic disease can be contagious as we mirror each other's wrong lifestyle choices, health also can be contagious! Given half a chance, our bodies will heal themselves.[6]

THE FOUR COMPONENTS OF GOOD HEALTH

The following four components are key to focus on for better health.

* **Drink:** plenty of water
* **Move:** purposeful movement 30 minutes a day
* **Eat:** whole, clean foods
* **Sleep:** seven to eight hours each night

For many years, I knew these four components were important. What I didn't know was the how and why. Once I got an understanding of the impact of my choices in each of these four components, I was on my path toward excellent health.

If you are able to focus on making improvements in those four components as we'll talk about in this book, you will begin to notice a change in your health in just two weeks. And, you don't need to do all of these at once. Focus on one at a time. When those changes become part of your normal routine, add another change. It's your journey. It's the progress that's most important.

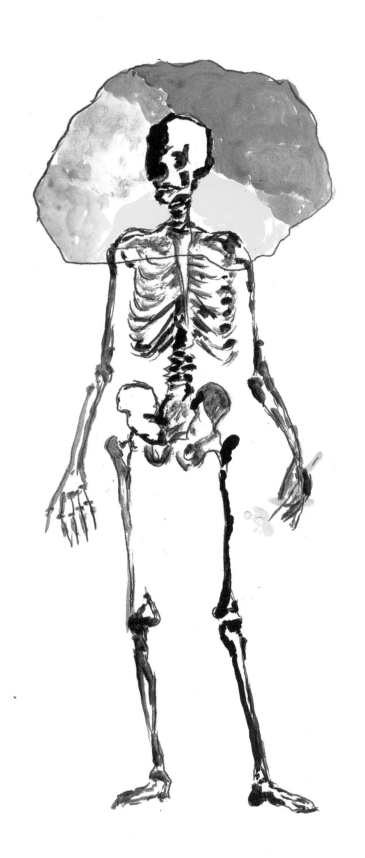

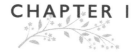

CHAPTER I

Body Systems

THIS IS YOUR ONE PRECIOUS LIFE. How are you going to "operate" it?

Your body is amazing. You have 78 organs in your body. They form 11 important organ systems[1] that work in concert. This is called connectivity of your body system.[2] Amazingly, they're also able to work independently when necessary.

The connectivity of our body systems seems to get lost in the Western Medicine model of specialists. It's hard to find a general practitioner anymore, even though we have abundant technology to support their value.

Your organ systems are:

* Cardiovascular/circulatory
* Digestive
* Endocrine
* Lymphatic
* Muscular
* Nervous

* Reproductive
* Respiratory
* Skin
* Skeletal
* Urinary/excretory

Western Medicine and its advances have definitely played a huge role in some critical health areas such as infectious diseases, transplants, and critical/acute events. Where Western Medicine seems to have lost its vision is in the connection of our various systems for overall and long-term wellness. Our body systems can work independently or interdependently. However, their ability to work *at all* depends on having a healthy environment.

How do you cultivate the healthy environment your body systems need to thrive?

Sally's Story

I remember when my mother, late in life, was taking 15 different medications, many of which were prescribed to offset the side effects of the other medications. My mother was never sure if she would be experiencing diarrhea or constipation. The uncertainty was stressful for her and physically exhausting.

Unfortunately, at that time in my mother's life, I was just beginning to understand herbs and medicines. When I requested information about the medications my mother was taking, I was overwhelmed by the pages of text that the druggist gave me. And, I certainly was overwhelmed by the format in which this information was presented.

Over time, I learned that the body is able to process at most five medications at a time. My mother being prescribed three times that amount for her little body was inappropriate—and certainly not healthy caring.

Take a moment to think about the following statistics that were presented in an Institute for Integrative Nutrition (IIN) lecture by Libby Weaver, PhD, internationally acclaimed nutritional biochemist.[3]

* Your body has approximately 50 trillion cells (To put that into perspective: 1 million seconds equal 12 days. 1 trillion seconds equals 32,000 years.)

* Every second, each cell in your body coordinates billions of chemical reactions.

* Your heart beats 100,000 times a day. Multiply your age times 365 times 100,000 to calculate how many beats your heart has made to date.

* Your heart pumps 7,500 liters of blood through 96,000 vessels.

* Every month, you completely regenerate your outer layer of skin.

What an amazing organism! I know that I need to reboot my computer every few days. I get a "servicing" on the computer every quarter, and I'm lucky if I have a functioning CPU for 3 years.

Yet, I seldom see a doctor, even with all the miles I have! Since my thirties, I have aspired to have good health. Sometimes my focus was exercise;

other times it was diet. It wasn't until my mid-fifties that I realized that I needed to make these two a part of my life, not just a short-term solution. However, in my late sixties, I learned how to fix my food choices, and then, my weight struggles also disappeared.

Of your body's 11 organ systems, we're going to focus on four here: digestive, cardiovascular, respiratory, and immune including lymph. Why focus on these? I found these to be the basic systems that influence our state of health. Unfortunately, we take them for granted until a problem occurs. Therefore, I thought that a better understanding of these core systems should help prevent some major problems.

DIGESTIVE SYSTEM

"It is pretty amazing when you reflect upon it (digestion) that you can sit at a dinner party enjoying yourself extravagantly—eating, talking, laughing, breathing, slurping wine—and that your naso-pharyngeal guardians will send everything to the right place, in two directions, without you having to give it a moment's consideration...while you are chattering away about work or school catchment zones or the price of kale, your brain is closely monitoring not just the taste and freshness of what you are eating but also its bulk and texture. So, it will allow you to swallow a large "wet" abolishing (like oyster or lump of ice cream) but insists on a more meticulous chewing for small, dry, sharp items like nuts and seeds that might not pass so smoothly."

—*The Body* BY BILL BRYSON[4]

Digestion is the processing system to feed our bodies. It starts with our thoughts of eating, which start the saliva and gastric juices flowing. Gut health affects mood, immune response, and predisposition to weight gain.

Components of the Digestive System

* Brain: You see the food, smell it, and think your intention to eat.
* Mouth: You chew the food completely, and your saliva begins the digestive process.

* Throat: It's a conduit with many roles, moving air, food, and liquid.

* Stomach: Here you mix and grind food through gastric juices to pass on to your small intestine.

* Small intestine: Your food is further digested, and nutrients and minerals are absorbed.

* Liver: This organ processes the nutrients absorbed from your small intestine.

* Large intestine: This stage converts food waste into feces, absorbs essential vitamins produced by gut bacteria, and reclaims water from feces.

Phases of Digestion and Role of Each Phase

* Oral phase: Food is chewed well, and saliva—liquid "gold"—starts the food breakdown.

* Gastric phase: In this phase, food is broken down into food molecules. The smaller the food pieces are that enter the stomach, the more efficient the gastric phase can be. So, chew your food well. The acid in your stomach is a defense system. Gastric acids prevent salmonella, parasites, and yeast mold by neutralizing it. A gastric fluid pH of 1 to 2 is deleterious to many microbial pathogens. (Normal body pH is 7.4.)

* Intestinal phase: The first part of this phase, which occurs in your small intestine, is where 90 percent of nutrients are digested and absorbed. The intestines also play a critical role in the development of white blood cells, which are your immune soldiers.

DID YOU KNOW

The cells that line the intestinal wall are only one layer of tightly fitted cells—like puzzle pieces. A break or opening in the wall may lead to leaky gut syndrome, allowing bacteria and other toxins to leak into the blood system.

The second part of the intestinal phase occurs in your large intestine, which absorbs water to eliminate waste. Your large intestine is the home to microflora, fights infestations, enhances nature to absorption, and promotes optimal bowel movements (transit time).

Microflora is a term used to describe the bacteria in your intestines. When this bacteria is healthy, it can provide some of these beneficial tasks: aid digestion, manufacture nutrients, protect against food-borne pathogens, and maybe help regulate body weight. However, poor nutrition and drugs impact the health of these bacteria.

How long does it take for your body to complete these phases of digestion? The bowel transit time—or the time it takes for food to travel from your mouth to the end of your large intestine—varies, even in the same person. The average transit time of food through the colon is 12 to 24 hours. Someone who is constipated would experience longer transit time. The longer food takes to pass through the colon, the more harmful bacterial degradation products are produced.

Your Turn

What's your body's transit time? Eat corn or red beets and monitor how long after eating they show up in a bowel movement.

FOOD EATEN: _____

DATE/TIME EATEN: _____

DATE/TIME PASSED: _____

KEY COMPONENTS OF DIGESTION

Let's look more closely at two important components of digestion, which are often taken for granted—your mouth and gastric acid.

The Mouth

This is the mechanical part of the digestive process, or maceration, the chewing of your food. The more that your food is broken down, the easier it is for your stomach to accept and process.

In your mouth, you have 12 salivary glands that over your lifetime will secrete around 31,700 quarts.[5] Chewing stimulates your salivary glands to release enzymes. The more you chew your food, the more enzymes get mixed into the composition. Chewing your food well is a first line of defense against disease—even cancer.[6] Did your mom tell you to "chew every bite 20 times?" This is a good rule of thumb for both breaking down food and mixing the enzymes.

Your teeth and tongue are the most familiar aspects in our maceration process. We have four types of teeth, for four separate purposes:

* Incisors bite into food
* Canines tear food apart
* Pre-molars tear and crush food
* Molars grind, tear, and crush food.[7]

The thin coat of enamel on your teeth is the hardest substance in your body. Although it's hard, it's also fragile: Once it's gone, it can't regenerate. That's why it's so important to have good dental health and have cavities filled once found.

When you think about the chewing power of your teeth, isn't it amazing that when you bite your tongue or cheek, it's usually only a temporary injury?

Gastric Acid

The acidity of your primary digestive juice, hydrochloric acid (HCL), can dissolve metal.[8] As we age, the acidity tends to lessen, which can cause inefficient digestion in the stomach and also impacting the enzyme production of your liver, pancreas, and small intestine.

You can enhance your HCL production by taking an herbal bitters tonic, such as a compound with fresh dandelion root, fresh artichoke leaf, gentian root, fresh peppermint herb, Angelica root, and orange peel.[9] In addition to increasing HCL production, bitters also increase saliva flow, increase bile in liver, and stimulate the production of small intestine and gastric juices. All of this benefits the goal of digestion: the absorption of nutrients into your circulatory system.

Sally's Story

Through my herbal and nutrition training, I learned that acid reflux should first be addressed by using bitters. What we think of as having too much stomach acid may actually be having too little.

After you have finished eating, it takes about an hour for your stomach to digest your food. One way to make your digestion more efficient is to restrict beverage intake about 30 minutes before eating and 60 minutes after eating. This helps with digestion because fluids deplete the effectiveness of gastric acid. The lower the pH, the stronger the gastric acid; beverages will weaken this pH factor.

Relationship of the Digestive System to Other Systems

After your digestive system extracts the nutrients from the food you eat, it relies on another system to get those nutrients to where they need to go. The digestive system works very closely with your circulatory system to get the absorbed nutrients distributed throughout your body. The circulatory system also carries chemical signals from your endocrine system that control the speed of digestion.

The digestive system also works in parallel with your excretory system, which is composed of your kidneys and bladder. While the digestive system collects and removes undigested solids, the excretory system filters compounds from the bloodstream and collects them in urine. These two systems are closely connected in controlling the amount of water in your body.[10]

Top Tips for a Healthy Digestive System

* Eat real food, such as legumes, nuts and seeds, whole grains, colorful fruits, and a variety of vegetables.

* Limit processed foods. Their additives can hinder digestion, including trans fats (hydrogenated oils), high fructose corn syrup (HFCS), artificial sweeteners (sucralose, aspartame, and saccharine), and artificial colors.

* Get plenty of fiber, including both soluble fiber (such as black beans, lima beans, avocados, Brussel sprouts, sweet potatoes, and broccoli) and insoluble fiber (such as wheat bran, whole grains, nuts/seeds, and skins of fruits and vegetables).

* Add prebiotics, which are found in fruits and vegetables.

* Eat healthy fats, such as monounsaturated fats, which are found in olive oil, canola oil, peanut oil, sesame oil, and avocado oil. Avoid trans fats, which are chemically altered fats.

* Stay hydrated by drinking plenty of water.

* Manage stress. Stress hormones directly affect digestion.

* Eat mindfully: Sit down, relax, turn off the TV.

* Chew your food well.

* Don't eat too fast; slow down.

* Don't overeat.

* Get moving. Regular exercise is beneficial to digestion—especially after a meal.[11]

Signs of Improper Digestion

* Chronic constipation

* Food intolerance, such as gas, bloating, heartburn, and headache

* Gastroesophageal reflux disease (GERD) – heartburn

* Inflammatory bowel disease, such as Crohn's disease and ulcerative colitis[12]

Quick Note about Sugar

Some health professionals liken the effects of pure, cane sugar to that of co-caine—very addictive. Perhaps you're fortunate in that eating one cookie is sufficient. That was not my case. It always took me a couple of cookies or candies to somewhat satisfy my craving.

Our bodies seek monosaccharides: simple sugars, consisting of one sugar unit that can't be further broken down. Glucose, fructose, and galactose are all simple sugars and important in nutrition. Foods with healthy sugars include fresh fruit (not dried or juice), carrots, beets, and sweet potatoes.

If the ingested sugar is not one the body can easily metabolize in the liver—such as fructose syrup, corn syrup, and cane sugar found in manufactured desserts, treats, and soda—then it's not used in the body for energy. Instead, it's stored as fat.

I've learned to substitute other sweeteners for cane sugar, such as coconut palm sugar, maple syrup, agave nectar, and honey. They may provide a greater sweet taste than cane sugar, so you may want to experiment with this conversion in your recipes.

I cup cane sugar equals:

* ¾ cup agave nectar and lower oven temperature 25°F
* ¾ cup honey and lower oven temperature 25°F
* ¾ cup maple syrup plus I teaspoon baking soda
* I cup coconut palm sugar

When reading a product label, remember that natural sugars exist within whole foods. Added sugars are introduced in the processing. Added sugars provide no nutritional value, and they will spike the body's blood sugar levels.

Your Turn

If you think that a food may be causing digestive problems, you can take a simple test. If a food causes discomfort within three days of eating and occurs consistently on three separate occasions, you may want to eliminate it from your diet.

CARDIOVASCULAR/CIRCULATORY SYSTEM

"Anything that damages blood flow, damages and ages our brain. Our brains don't have to deteriorate. Think of a grape that becomes a raisin."

—DANIEL AMEN, MD[13]

The heart is the pump for the blood, which travels in this closed system of vessels. As a closed system, the blood continues to circulate throughout the vessels, carrying oxygen and nutrients as well as carbon dioxide and cell waste products.

Components of the Cardiovascular System

The primary components are:

* Heart: About the size of your fist, this muscular organ pumps blood throughout your body.
* Arteries: These vessels carry the oxygen rich blood to the body organs.
* Veins: These vessels carry deoxygenated blood from parts of the body back to the heart.
* Capillaries: The smallest of blood vessels, they carry and distribute oxygenated blood from arteries to the tissues of the body and deoxygenated blood from the tissues back into the veins

It's estimated that the average heart pumps more than five liters of blood every minute, even while you're at rest. This system is critical to maintaining the body's balance or homeostasis.[14,15]

Relationship of the Cardiovascular System to Other Systems

Your circulatory system interacts with every organ and system in your body. Every cell that needs oxygen needs access to the fluids in your circulatory system. The circulatory system and its fluids are super important to your digestive system that has absorbed nutrients from your food. It's also responsible for transporting oxygen to all cells and helping eliminate carbon dioxide waste. Hormones created in the endocrine system are also transported through the circulatory system.[16]

Top Tips for a Healthy Circulatory System

Each day:

* Eat real food, not processed food.
* Get regular exercise; for heart health get at least 30 minutes each day.
* Stay hydrated; it helps your heart to pump more easily.
* Practice deep breathing, which is good for your heart, circulation, and mind and for stress reduction—four benefits in one!

Additionally, the following activities should be included on a regular basis:[17]

* Maintain a healthy weight
* Cut down on salt
* Quit smoking
* Stay positive

Signs of Improper Cardiovascular System

* Chest pain: insufficient blood flow to the heart angina pectoris
* Abnormal rhythm: Arrhythmia
* Insufficient oxygen in the blood: Ischemia
* Hardening of the arteries: too much fat, arthrosclerosis
* Heart attack: insufficient blood flow in the heart mitral prolapse, stenosis[18, 19]

Your Turn

How do you determine your ideal body weight?

A popular and easy equation to use is the Hamwi equation, which was developed by Dr. G.J Hamwi:[20]

FOR WOMEN:

5 feet ideal weight is 100 pounds

• for each inch above 5 feet, add 5 pounds

• for each inch below 5 feet, subtract 5 pounds

My height: _____

Number of inches above 5 feet:

_____

Multiply number of inches above X 5 pounds: _____

Your ideal weight: 100 pounds + above = _____

FOR MEN:

5 feet ideal weight is 106 pounds

• for each inch above 5 feet, add 6 pounds

• for each inch below 5 feet, subtract 6 pounds

My height: _____

Number of inches above 5 feet:

_____

Multiply number of inches above X 6 pounds: _____

Your ideal weight: 106 pounds + above = _____

RESPIRATORY SYSTEM

The human body needs oxygen to sustain itself. According to the National Institute of Neurological Disorders and Stroke, after only about five minutes without oxygen, brain cells begin dying, which can lead to brain damage and death. [21]

Your respiratory system's primary function is the exchange of oxygen and carbon dioxide in the body. Its other functions include:

* Participation in the acid-base balance of the body: It can adjust the blood pH upward in minutes by exhaling CO_2 from the body.

* Phonation: Producing speaking sounds

* Pulmonary defense: This is the tiny muscular, hair-like projections on the cells (cilia) that line the airway.

* Metabolism: Removal of waste products (along with circulatory system) that occur from metabolism

Components of the Respiratory System

* Nose and nasal cavity support three primary functions:

  * Warm, moisten, and purify inspired air
  * Olfaction
  * Resonance, i.e. changes quality of voice

* Mouth: We have several options for breathing: through the mouth, nose, or both. Through the nose is the preferred option for our bodies because this type of breathing helps clean the sinus surface of pollen, dander, and dust. It also warms the air as you breathe it in. Did you ever inhale cold winter air through your mouth? Thank goodness for options. How could we breathe when we have colds without using our mouths?

* Pharynx: This is the passageway for air going to the lungs—and also for food on its way to the stomach.[23]

* Larynx: This organ allows air to pass through it, while keeping food and drink from blocking the airway.[24]

* Trachea: Commonly known as your windpipe, this provides air flow to and from the lungs for respiration.[25]

* Bronchi: These extensions of the windpipe shuttle air to and from the lungs.[26]

* Lungs: It's in your lungs where the gas is exchanged: oxygen for carbon dioxide.

* Alveoli: Tiny sacs within your lungs allow oxygen and carbon dioxide to move between your lungs and bloodstream.[27]

DID YOU KNOW

Smell is considered to be the most powerful of our five senses as it is closely linked with memory.[22] We can distinguish more than 10,000 scents. And, smell has a direct connection to the brain.

When we inhale, we take air/oxygen into our lungs. When we exhale, we eliminate carbon dioxide. The process of taking air into the lungs is inspiration or inhalation and the process of breathing it out is expiration or exhalation.[28] On average our lungs pump 13 pints of air every minute.[29]

Relationship of the Respiratory System to Other Systems

Your lungs work with your circulatory system to pump oxygen-rich blood to all cells in the body. The blood then collects carbon dioxide, and other waste products and transports them back to the lungs, where they're pumped out of the body when we exhale.[30]

Top Tips for a Healthy Respiratory System

* Stop smoking.

* Stay away from secondhand smoke.

* Avoid indoor and outdoor air pollution. According to the EPA, sources of indoor pollution include household cleaning products; newly installed flooring, upholstery, or carpet; paint; central HVAC; carbon monoxide; and radon. Indoor plants are a great way to help support indoor air quality.

* Avoid exposure to people who have the flu or viral infections.

* Exercise regularly.[31]

TopTip

It's important to exercise most days. Why? If you don't exercise your lung capacity regularly, your body will begin to adapt to a lower capacity which then leads to shortness of breath. A good deep breathing exercise done periodically throughout the day will be beneficial, for lung capacity and also for stress and mind clearing.

* Eat a healthy, balanced diet.

* Maintain a healthy weight. Excess fat increases pulmonary resistance and reduces respiratory muscle strength.

* Have an annual physical. It's important for lung health because it identifies respiration rate and can be a signal should the rate be less than 12 to 16 breathes per minute.

Signs of Improper Respiratory System[32]

Diseases and conditions of the respiratory system fall into two categories:

* Infections, such as influenza, bacterial pneumonia, and enterovirus respiratory virus, which is a virus that enters through the gastrointestinal tract and can affect the nervous system and has impact on respiratory secretions saliva and mucus:

  * Many lung infections are viral, which means they are caused by viruses, not bacteria. Antibiotics are effective against bacteria, but not viruses. According to Neal Chaisson, MD,[33] who practices pulmonary medicine at the Cleveland Clinic, there's not much that can be done for viral infections but to let them run their course. Antibiotics are not effective in treating viruses, and the best thing to do is just rest.

* Chronic diseases, such as asthma, chronic obstructive pulmonary disease (COPD), and lung cancer:

  * Asthma, which can be related to air pollution, tobacco smoke, factory fumes, cleaning solvents, pollution, foods, cold air, exercise, chemicals, and medications

  * Chronic Obstructive Pulmonary Disease (COPD): Cigarette smoking is the leading cause; however, other irritants such as pollution, chemical fumes, or dust can cause it as well. (This is especially inorganic chemical dust, which people are primarily exposed to through occupations. However, any airborne dust, moved through blowing or compressed air force versus vacuuming, including home dust can be an irritant to the lungs.)

* Lung cancer: causes include smoking, family history, and exposure to secondhand smoke, radon gas, and asbestos

LYMPH SYSTEM

Your lymph system is your extensive drainage system.

Although there are three primary functions for the lymph system, most of us are aware of its work in the immune function. It's your defense system against invading microorganisms and infections.

However, there are two other important functions:

* Detoxification/fluid balance: The lymph system returns the excess interstitial fluid (fluid that surrounds cells) back to the blood. Approximately 90 percent of this fluid can be returned. The rest goes to the capillaries, where it becomes a part of the interstitial fluid that surrounds the cell tissue.

* Nutrient absorption: The lymph system absorbs fats and fat-soluble vitamins, such as vitamin D, from the digestive system.

The lymph system moves fluid all over your body. However, your lymph system has no pump, unlike your circulatory system, which has your heart. This system relies on your activities to make it work: your skeletal muscle movements, respiratory movements, and contraction of smooth muscle in vessel walls.

Components of the Lymph System

* Lymph nodes: These small, bean-like structures filter and carry nutrients, lymph fluid, and waste.

* Tonsils: These are your first line of defense against infection in the throat.

The Immune System

Let's take a brief look at another system, the immune system.

When we think about the immune system, we often focus on germs and the lymph system, a very important part of our immune operation. Did you ever think that these items also contribute to the immune system—earwax, skin, tears? According to Bill Bryson in his book *The Body*, many of our immune cells have multiple jobs. One example provided in his book is that Interleukin-1 "not only attacks pathogens but also plays a role in sleep, which may go some way to explaining why we are so often drowsy when unwell."[34]

A little further he goes on to note that our immune system not only deals with germs, "it also has to respond to toxins, drugs, cancer cells, foreign objects and even your own state of mind." (stress, exhaustion)[35]

* Spleen: This organ filters out worn out red blood cells and other foreign bodies, such as germs.

* Thymus: This is the main organ in your lymph system. It "teaches" a subgroup of t-cells the difference between your body's own cells and alien cells. Examples of alien cells include foreign microorganisms, which can be bacteria or viruses.

All lymph organs carry high concentrations of white blood cells that identify and destroy toxins. [36]

Relationship of the Lymph System to Other Systems

Your lymph system works with your brain to keep a healthy fluid balance. It works with your cardiovascular system through the transporting of excessive tissue fluid from interstitial spaces throughout the body back to the blood stream. It also works with your digestive system by helping to absorb fats (lipids) and fat-soluble vitamins.

Top Tips for a Healthy Lymph System

Maintaining a healthy lymphatic system is important to prevent illness and keep other important body systems functioning. Encourage proper function of your lymphatic system by incorporating these healthy lifestyle tips:

* Drink plenty of water. The best water to drink is alkaline water followed by distilled water. (See page 44.)

* Eat a healthy diet rich in alkaline foods and vegetables that provide a full range of vitamins, minerals, and nutrients. Alkaline foods include leafy green vegetables, root vegetables, onion, garlic, ginger, and seasonal fruits. Why is eating in season important for your lymph system? Seasonal fruits and vegetables retain more of their nutrients than their counterparts providing more micronutrients.

* Include healthy fats in your diet by eating foods such as avocados, dark chocolate, whole eggs, fatty fish, and extra virgin olive oil.

* Exercise daily, including both aerobic activity such as walking, running, cycling, swimming, or boxing and anaerobic physical activity, such as weight-lifting, sprints, isometrics, and high intensity interval training.

* Avoid pollutants, toxic substances, and unhealthy environments. These pollutants tax the lymph system and thereby impact its ability to help other systems function properly.

* Learn to manage stress through techniques such as yoga, meditation, and exercise to promote wellness.

* Have a massage, which helps to move lymph fluid.[37]

Having a massage? Make sure to drink water after a massage because it will help with the detoxification.

TopTip

Signs of Improper Lymph System

Your lymphatic system is constantly working to keep your body balanced. Maintaining its health is important for its own role and also for the role it plays in many other body systems.[38] Some of the signs that lymphatic fluid is not moving effectively and that toxins may be building up in your body are:

* Fatigue
* Swollen glands
* Puffiness in eyes or face
* Swelling in the fingers (tight rings) or ankles
* Bloating or holding on to water
* Headaches
* Sinus infections
* Skin issues, such as dry or itchy skin
* Soreness or stiffness upon waking
* Constipation
* Weight gain and extra belly fat
* Breast swelling or tenderness
* Fogginess in the brain
* Worsened allergies
* Food sensitivities
* Increased colds or flu

Sally's Story

Recently I had a bout with food poisoning. I was amazed at how quickly the immune response came on as I felt and heard my stomach reacting. As the day progressed, I could almost feel the immune defense working its way through my digestive system. After about 18 hours, it must have made the "all clear" message because I could finally look at food again!

OPTIMIZING YOUR BODY SYSTEM WELLNESS

In addition to the tips listed for each body system, to reach and maintain a level of wellness, you also need to have intention (directed impulse of conscientiousness of what we aim to create) and gratitude (awareness and appreciation) in your life. To do this, your mind and body need to work together. Things that you ignore will not go away.

Two important things to watch for as clues your body systems are not well are pain and inflammation. Let's talk about each in turn.

Pain: The Body's Alert System

When we have pain, it's a warning signal that your body is trying to get your attention. Our bodies are always trying to tell us the reason behind what's happening. Unfortunately, due to the marketing dollars spent by the food industry and pharmaceutical firms, we often only listen with our head and forget the body.

Our bodies tend to cluster ailments. Pay attention to the region in which you are experiencing the discomfort—not just the body organ. Then ask yourself: What else could be going on?

The next time that you are not feeling 100 percent, ask yourself a few questions:

* Where is the pain or hurt located?

* What other systems or organs are in this same area?

* Did I do anything differently (eat, exercise) that might have caused this?

* Am I hydrated?

* Am I comfortable enough to work through and listen or is a physician visit warranted?

An easy example is a food craving. Tastes craved can often give insights into problems. Cravings many times relate to the body's need for water. So why not consider a glass of water before giving in to that piece of pie or cake?

Inflammation: The Body's Subtle Cry for Help

Before leaving this section, I wanted to spend a few paragraphs on the importance of understanding inflammation. Researchers have linked inflammation to nearly every critical disease of aging—in every single organ system. Reduce inflammation, and you can clear a path to a happier, healthier, longer life.[39]

But first, there is a bit of good news on inflammation. Inflammation is our life saver in that it allows us to fend off various disease related bacteria, viruses, and parasites. The instant any of these bad guys slips into the body, inflammation pulls together a defensive attack that lays waste to both invader and infected tissue.

However, as quickly as inflammation responds or turns on, it should

Sally's Story

At the first sign of a cold or flu, I start taking raw garlic, which is a great antiviral and antibacterial.

To take garlic, I first cut the clove into small pieces. Then I either put the pieces on a piece of bread – garlic bread! Or I stir the garlic pieces into a teaspoon of honey.

The raw, uncooked essential oil in garlic is where the action is. That's why it's important to chew this mixture while in your mouth to release the essential oils.

Note that garlic is a blood thinner, so if you are on blood thinning medication, don't try this remedy without your doctor's permission. Eating raw garlic by itself can turn one's stomach upside down. That's why I eat it with bread or honey.

then turn off. If not, if instead inflammation becomes long-term and chronic, that's when it becomes a problem.

Sometimes the on/off switch doesn't work. It could be genetic-related, but often lifestyle habits like smoking or high blood pressure will keep the switch on. This is when our bodies begin to experience extended periods of inflammation, leading to the potential of a chronic stress situation.

There are two types of inflammation caused by stress: acute and chronic.

Acute Inflammation

Acute inflammation is the body's response to an event that puts the body on a short-term high alert. These events include cut, cold, sprained, and exercised muscles. It's important that after the event is addressed, the high alert switch goes off.

Chronic Inflammation

Chronic inflammation is continual inflammation within the body. This is what happens when the "off switch" doesn't seem to work. A continual low-grade inflammation can lead to the destruction of healthy cells. Unfortunately, a low-grade inflammation is gradual and generally not noticeable until it leads to a chronic condition, such as heart disease, diabetes, arthritis, and experts believe even Alzheimer's disease.[40]

The states of immune response are the following:

Alarm state: Your body is in panic mode, and this is the activation of the body's response to the event.

Adaptive state: After the initial inflammation response, your body returns to homeostasis.

Extended release state: If the event continues, the inflammation doesn't go away. This lowers your immunity, increases your blood pressure and heart rate, impacts your mood, makes it more difficult to sleep, and increases fat storage.

Exhaustive or chronic state: The event and inflammation have continued for so long that your body isn't able to return to the rest state.

Events and circumstances that can cause low-grade inflammation include:

* Lack of exercise
* Carrying extra weight
* A sudden change in weight
* Poor eating
* Drinking excessive alcohol
* Smoking
* Always feeling agitated
* Feeling stressed

A presentation by Arianna Huffington of *The Huffington Post* that I attended noted several studies on the effects of stress:

* University of Miami: Stress fuels cancer.[41]
* Yale University: Stress shrinks the brain.[42]
* *Journal of Molecular Psychology*: Stress prematurely ages children.[43]
* Mayo Clinic: Stress spurs depressive symptoms.[44]
* Pennsylvania State University: Stress increases the risk of chronic disease.[45]

Studies show that chronic stress decreases the effectiveness of the immune system, which can result in more colds and illness, as well as increased weight. Here are some ways to counter stress.

* Engage in calming activities, such as meditation, tai chi, yoga, and deep breathing.
* Keep an organized environment. Make both your home and work clutter free and peaceful.
* Plan, schedule, and prioritize tasks. You can still deviate from your plans. Situations change, and you need to be able to adapt.
* Delegate wherever possible. At home, it helps with character development of children and increases support from your spouse. At work, it helps to build your "bench" strength; increase the number of others who can help you, training others to do tasks that you would normally assume.
* Make better food choices, eating more whole food, less processed foods, and more fruits and vegetables—seasonal and organic, when possible.

Sally's Story

Although I consider myself to be fairly balanced, whenever I get a body massage, the therapist finds my adrenal glands to be in overload.

Adrenal glands are the size of small walnuts and located at the top of each kidney. They are hormone-producing glands, and they manufacture and secrete 505 hormones. The adrenal glands' manufacturing of the hormones helps to balance the body's stress reaction.

A good body massage includes reflexology. In reflexology, the link to the adrenals is in the arch of your foot. When the therapist begins a pressure massage here, I almost fly off the table. Fortunately, with a more regular routine of massage, this is getting less sensitive. My adrenal glands are seemingly less stressed.

* Listen to your body systems. Don't let your head take the lead. Control your inner voice; this voice inside your head isn't you because you are listening to it. Turn down the volume (and the propaganda). Reboot through silence, breathing, and eye gazing[46], which is similar to daydreaming: looking into the distance without any specific focus.

* Do all things in moderation. Extremism in any form—diet, herbs, drugs, religion, lifestyle, etc.—will always tip your ability to be balanced. Just because one pill might alleviate a headache doesn't mean that you should take several!

* Visualize elements of your life balance or homeostasis as a seesaw. For example, if you are in balance, your exercise is balanced out by your rest. You're in balance when the seesaw is level or in the middle. However, there might be times when you're up in the air, or your partner is up in the air. Your relationship is out of balance. We need to strive for being in that middle zone in all areas of life for wellness.

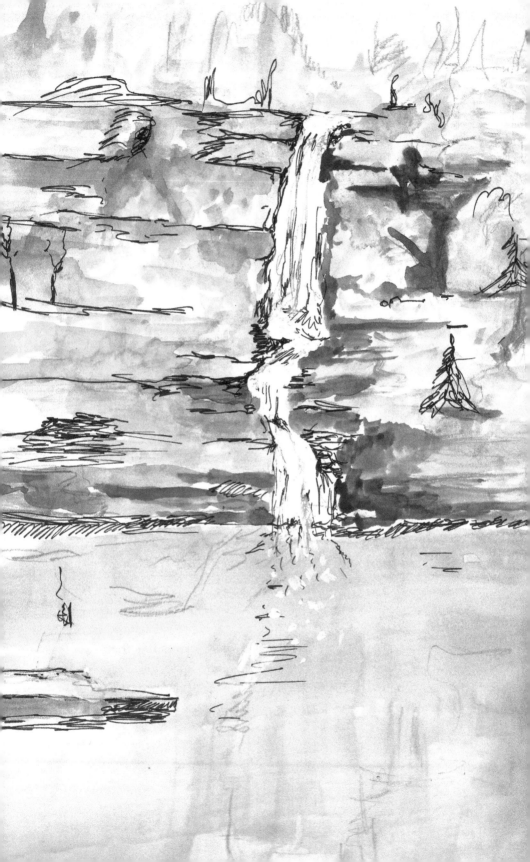

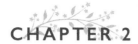

CHAPTER 2

Drink

WATER IS ESSENTIAL FOR ALL LIFE. Water makes up more than 70 percent of our earth's surface; however, only 2.5 percent is fresh water. Plants, wildlife, and humans all need water. In fact, adult bodies are comprised of approximately 60 percent water.

Our sense of thirst diminishes with age. Therefore, there may be fewer triggers to encourage us to drink water.

Without water, humans can survive only three to five days, whereas we can survive without food for almost three weeks. Fortunately, food can provide about 20 percent of our water needs, so our need for drinking water is lessened. However, we do need to balance our intake with the daily loss of water through sweating, exhaling, and urinating. Without the additional 80 percent from drinking water, dehydration begins to occur.

Our bodies are so well designed that when our cells need water that they aren't getting, they want to protect critical organs, such as the heart and brain. Therefore, cells in your extremities and less-essential organs reduce their water needs to support the critical functions.

Did you ever notice those prune-looking ridges that your fingertips get when you haven't had sufficient water intake? That's an early warning sign of dehydration.[1]

Water dictates the shape of other molecules. Everything under our skin works in water, and it should move and not be stagnant. Water plays a key role in the transportation of nutrients, removal of water products, regulation of cellular volume, and control of temperature.

IMPORTANCE OF WATER

Here are some of the ways that maintaining a proper hydration level supports your body.[2]

* Forms proper amounts of saliva for digestion
* Keeps mucosal membranes moist
* Supports cell growth, reproduction, and survival
* Flushes body waste
* Lubricates joints
* Supports your brain's manufacturing of hormones and neurotransmitters
* Regulates body temperature
* Acts as a shock absorber for your brain and spinal cord
* Converts food to components needed for survival
* Helps deliver oxygen throughout the body

The following situations may require us to have an increased need for water.

* Illness
* Fever
* Diarrhea
* High altitudes
* Infections, such as bladder or urinary
* Excessive alcohol consumption

Sally's Story

As my father aged, I noticed his fingertips looking like prunes. I would suggest that he drink more water, and he would retort that it would only make him urinate more. Instead, he would drink iced tea, but no water. My dad didn't understand that the iced tea couldn't fulfill his body's hydration needs. Nor did he understand that drinking more water wouldn't make his trips to the bathroom more frequent. He also had several urinary tract infections, which can be triggered by dehydration.

Your body will need more water during the day than at night. To limit your night excursions to the bathroom, you may want to stop active water drinking an hour or two before sleep. Keeping a glass of water by your bed might be good for the occasional coughing needs as well as to be your first water intake in the morning.

We often confuse our body's need for water with food, thinking we're hungry when we're actually thirsty. Our signals get crossed. That's why diet advisors suggest drinking a glass of water before eating a snack and 30 minutes before each meal. As a bonus, this helps to maintain a healthy weight!

Your Turn

How much water do you need? According to most research, adult males need about 3 liters (3.2 quarts or 102 ounces) per day. With 20 percent being provided through food, that would equate to about 10 cups (8 ounces) of water each day. Adult females need about 2.3 liters (9.5 cups) of which 7.5 -8 ounce-cups would be supplied by drinking water. Please note, that these are average figures. Your needs will vary based on height, weight, activity levels, and age.[3]

There are several water calculators available on the internet. A basic approach to water needs, assuming limited activity, is to take your body weight and divide by 2, which gives you the number of ounces. Divide that by 8 for the number of cups.

If you are fairly active, then you may want to try the calculator.

If you are taking medication, it is important to check with your physician as to the recommended daily water amounts. According to the Cleveland Clinic, if you are taking pills, it is important to take them with a full glass of water. Not drinking a full 8 ounces might prevent the medication from working properly.

HOW MUCH WATER DO YOU NEED TO DRINK EACH DAY? _____

FOR A DAY, KEEP TRACK HOW MUCH YOU ACTUALLY DRINK: _____

HOW MANY OUNCES ARE YOU FALLING SHORT? _____

Consequences of a Lack of Water

According to physician and nutritionist Eddie Fatakhov, MD, "America is dehydrated, and that's a problem because 83 percent of your lungs are water. If you take the heart and the brain, 73 percent is water. If you take the bones, about 31 percent is water. If you take the kidneys and muscles, about 76 percent is water. Your body is made up of water."[4]

Here are some of the consequences of lack of water, also known as dehydration.

* Mood swings
* Dry skin
* Decreased cognitive function
* Headaches
* Fatigue

If dehydration is combined with heat exhaustion, a very critical life-threatening condition is reached. That's why it's especially important to be hydrated in hot weather.

Types of Water

There are so many choices of water these days. Which is the best? It mostly comes down to personal preference: What type of water will help you keep the level of hydration that you should have? As with most beverage and food choices, it's important for us to know the ingredients and keep the processing additives at a minimal level.

Tap water: If water is on a municipal system, it must adhere to the Environmental Protection Agency clean water standards. The Environmental

DID YOU KNOW

It's probably not a surprise that dehydration is a problem in hot weather. But did you know it's also a problem in cold weather? Cold weather tends to move body fluids from your extremities to your core, increasing your urine output and adding to dehydration. So, when you're in a cold climate, don't rely on thirst to tell you when you need to drink. Drink often—before you're thirsty.[5]

Sally's Story

In my early corporate career, I had a boss who always had a glass of water on her desk. Obviously, this made an impact on me as I still recall it; however, it didn't make me a convert.

Years later, when I had a kidney stone attack, I was told to increase my water intake, which I did often but not always. With my herbal and integrative nutrition learning, I became profoundly aware that I needed to consistently include water each day.

Now I keep a glass of water on my desk that holds about two cups, as well as a stainless-steel water bottle in my car and gym bag.

I wonder how different my body might be today if I had followed my boss's example all those years ago.

Working Group (EWG.org) recommends filtered tap water over bottled water.[6] Make sure to clean the aerator or removable part of the faucet.

Well water: If the water is on a well system, it's good to have the water checked periodically for chemicals and bacteria. Here, too, make sure to clean the aerator or removable part of the faucet.

Bottled water: Look for the source of the water and if provided in a plastic bottle, the bisphenol A (BPA) level. BPA is an industrial chemical that's been used to make certain plastics and resins since the 1960s. According to *Scientific America*, BPA free bottles might have a replacement industrial chemical that might also be hazardous.[7] Therefore, glass or stainless steel are the healthier options. If you buy filled plastic water bottles, don't reuse the empty bottles.

Spring water: This water is derived from an underground formation from which water flows naturally to the surface of the earth. Spring water must be collected only at the spring or through a borehole, tapping the underground formation feeding the spring.

Mineral water: This is natural water that has a constant level and relative proportions of mineral and trace elements, containing no less than 250 parts per million total of dissolved solids.

Sparkling water: This water is also known as sparkling mineral water, and it's found in natural springs. It's naturally carbonated due to the presence of various minerals. Note that it will still hydrate the body.

Artesian water: This water comes from a well that taps a specific layer of rock or sand.[8]

Carbonated water: This water contains dissolved carbon dioxide gas, either artificially injected under pressure or occurring due to natural geological processes. It will hydrate the body; however, it's best to drink plain water when hydrating due to exercise.

Seltzer: This water has artificial carbonation. It includes seltzer and club soda, and it's regulated like soda.[9]

Purified water: This water has been filtered or processed to remove impurities, such as chemicals, bacteria, algae, and other contaminants. It's usually produced using groundwater or tap water.[10]

Distilled water: This water has gone through the process of distillation to remove impurities. The water is boiled, steam is collected, which returns to the water upon cooling. This process removes more impurities than purified water.[11]

Drinking water should have a neutral pH of 7. (pH level is a measure of how acidic or basic water is.) Your body works best with a balanced pH of 7.4. Disruption of this balance in either direction can cause a condition (acidosis, alkalosis), requiring medical treatment.

Alkaline water has a higher pH level than tap water.

Acidic water exposes your body to heavy metals and minerals present in the water. Acidic water often causes problems for pipes, as it is highly corrosive and leads to damage.[12]

Water quality, regardless of how your home receives it (well or municipal) should be tested periodically, especially if the well is near farmed property or the house's infrastructure is old. There are companies that test water, in-home kits, and water service companies that can provide this support.

Here are some examples of water type labels:

Seltzer Label	Sparkling Water Label	Tonic Water Label
Calories 0	Calories 0	Calories 130
Total Fat 0 g	Total Fat 0 g	Total Fat 0
Sodium 5 mg	Sodium 0 mg	Sodium 55 mg
Total Carbs 0g	Total Carbs 0 g	Total Carbs 33 g
Protein 0g	Total sugars 0	Sugars 32 g
INGREDIENTS: carbonated water, natural flavor	Total added sugar 0	Protein 0 g
	INGREDIENTS: Carbonated water, natural flavors	**INGREDIENTS:** Carbonated water, High Fructose Corn Syrup, Citric Acid, Sodium Benzoate, Quinine, Natural Flavors

Hydration Impact of Other Beverages

Other beverages, such as coffee and tea, aren't water, and so they don't hydrate you like water. Here's the scoop on other beverages.

Caffeinated coffee and tea: According to the Mayo Clinic, coffee and tea with caffeine may have a mild diuretic affect, but they don't cause fluid loss in excess of volume ingested.[13] Recent research has debunked the coffee/tea dehydration myth. Although the caffeine won't negatively impact hydration, it can be a stress stimulator in your body. But both coffee and tea do offer health benefits. Be aware that added components, such as creamer and sweetener, can offset the health factors.

A black cup of coffee contains caffeine, which can improve energy levels, and nutrients, such as riboflavin, pantothenic acid, manganese, potassium, magnesium, and niacin.

Tea (white, green, or black) contains less caffeine than coffee, and depending on the type, provides health benefits of antioxidants. White tea is the less processed version, retaining more of the antioxidants.

Soda, fruit juice, and sport drinks: Sodas, even diet ones, have a bad reputation as lacking nutritional value, but they can still be hydrating. Juices and sports drinks are also hydrating. You can lower the sugar content by diluting them with water.[14]

Alcohol: Alcohol is a diuretic, and therefore, it can quickly dehydrate your body. Ever have the morning-after hangover? In most cases, the cause is dehydration by alcohol. Besides being conscientious of your intake, it's always good to drink water along with your wine, beer, or mixed drink. You may want to help offset any hangover potential by drinking water before going to sleep.[15]

Lemon water: Taken first thing in the morning as a warm drink, it can help to detox your system from all its overnight maintenance work.[17]

Food Sources of Water

Most people get around 20 percent of their water from food. Here's a list of the top food sources of water and their percentage of water.[18]

* Iceberg lettuce: 96 percent
* Radishes: 95 percent
* Celery: 95 percent
* Cucumber: 95 percent
* Tomatoes: 94 percent
* Zucchini: 94 percent
* Cabbage: 92 percent
* Cauliflower: 92 percent
* Spinach: 92 percent
* Strawberries: 91 percent
* Cantaloupe: 90 percent
* Bell pepper: 90 percent
* Peaches: 89 percent
* Oranges: 88 percent
* Grapefruit: 88 percent
* Cottage cheese: 80 percent
* Yogurt, plain: 75 percent

DID YOU KNOW

Lemon is an interesting juice. Outside of the body, it's acidic. But once lemon is fully digested, it becomes alkalizing, providing many health benefits.[18]

Lemons are a good source of vitamin C. Some evidence-based benefits provided by Healthline include:

* Heart health
* Help with weight control
* Prevention of kidney stones
* Digestive health

Tips to Drink More Water

It's challenging to make drinking eight to nine glasses of water a part of one's daily routine. However, here are some tips that the US Centers for Disease Control and Prevention offers.[19]

* Carry a water bottle with you throughout the day for easy access to water. I carry a 16-ounce, stainless steel bottle to the gym, in the car, in my brief bag. It's best to drink small amounts throughout the day.

* Choose water instead of sugar-sweetened beverages, even when eating out.

* Add a wedge of lime or lemon to water to help improve taste. You could also try other fruit in your water, such as apples or strawberries.

* Try chilling freezer-safe water bottles for easy access to ice-cold water throughout the day. Cold water might also help to burn more calories because the body needs to warm the water before it can use it.

According to Fereydoon Batmanghelidj, MD, an internationally renowned researcher, author and advocate of the natural healing power of water, at Watercure.com, when we get sick, most symptoms can be reduced by increased water consumption.[20]

Here are some ways you can help ensure quality water in your home.

* Purchase a water test kit for your home and test at least annually.
* Purchase eco-friendly water purifiers.

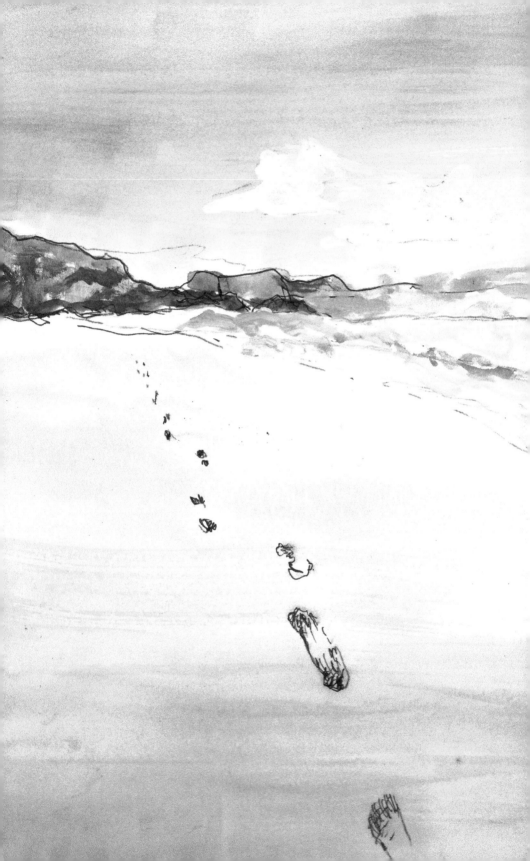

CHAPTER 3

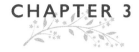

Move

TO MOVE OR NOT TO MOVE, should not be *your question.*

Exercise changes your body, and it also changes your mind, attitude, and mood.[1]

First, let's get on the same page with some definitions.

* Physical activity is any bodily movement produced by skeletal muscles that result in energy expenditure. Examples from daily life may include work-related movement, sports, physical conditioning, and housework.

* Exercise is a subset of physical activity that is planned, structured, and repetitive and has the objective of the improvement or maintenance of physical fitness.

* Physical fitness is a set of attributes that are either health or skill related.[2]

* Recreation is any activity done for enjoyment when one is not working. Recreating self, get it?[3]

The Importance of Exercise

As you age, it becomes extremely important to regularly move your muscles. Sedentary living is easy with our lives filled with helpers such as: remote controls, computers, and vehicles. However, our bodies weren't designed for sedentary living. Sitting is not healthy for our bodies.

How long do you want to live independently? As you age, exercise will help you remain independent longer by increasing your:

Strength: Your body's ability to use force. This involves the use of your back muscles and supports your ability to pull versus push, which is something we lose as we age.

Balance: Your body's ability to be centered and stable when shifting weight from side to side as in walking is important to prevent falls. For balance, your body relies heavily on strong gluts, hamstrings, and hip flexors.

Flexibility: Your body's ability for joint range of motion also helps you avoid falls. Flexibility provides stability. Especially important are flexible shoulders, knees, and pelvis.

Cardiovascular health: Your body's ability to efficiently use oxygen and exhale carbon dioxide by raising the heart rate helps to strengthen our muscles by increasing the capillary growth in the muscle.

These four areas are often taken for granted—until they are weak.

When we gave up the daily playground in elementary school, most of us began a path that led to becoming less active each day. When we entered the workforce, many of us became consumed by our jobs and then families, which meant even less time to exercise. This adult life became exhausting. How could we fit in exercise? We were already so tired!

Rather than trying to fit in exercise, we need to view purposeful movement or exercise as a part of our daily requirements. It's as important to your health as healthy meals, clean water, and mind- and mood-boosting productive work. Exercise is just as important to your health now as it was when you were growing up—maybe even more so. However, as grown-ups, we have such busy schedules that we have to schedule in our "play."

Benefits of Exercise

* Exercise provides stress. Although you might feel like exercise is an added stress, understand that this is a healthy stress.

* Exercise provides the release of hormones, such as cortisol, epinephrine,

DID YOU KNOW

Some experts consider sitting to be the new smoking! Being sedentary is that bad for your health.

Sally's Story

I came to truly understand the reality of the importance of exercise at age 58 when I read Younger Next Year *by Chris Crowley and Henry S. Lodge, MD.[4] It changed my life, literally. Sure, as a Phys Ed major in college (turned Parks and Rec) and an athlete, I should have known better. But I didn't. I enjoyed not running laps anymore and not having late afternoon workouts. Who knows where I would be today if I had just continued this moving in my thirties, forties, or early fifties. Regardless, this book spoke to me, and for the past 12 years, I have gotten younger each year!*

My energy levels have increased, and I have stayed true to incorporating exercise as a part of my daily routine. This along, with my nutrition changes, has gotten me to a weight that resembles my college years.

and neo-epinephrine. These are our three major stress hormones. Exercise allows the release in a "good stress" situation, not the usual "fight or flight" stress reaction.

* Working out offers the opportunity to "clear your head," which is extremely important in this age of technology disruption and 24/7 living.

* The breakdown of muscle that occurs when exercising leads to the building of new, stronger muscle. It's because of this breakdown that we need to alternate our exercise routine so that muscles get a rest.[4]

* It can help you look better by improving the look of your skin.

* Exercise helps to reduce the risk of infection because it strengthens your immune system.

* Exercise also decreases the risk of diabetes and insulin insensitivity and helps you reach and maintain a healthy weight.

* Moving your body creates stronger lung muscles by increasing oxygen and carbon dioxide exchange.

* It helps build bone density.

* It's good for your heart and strengthens your cardiovascular system, raises good cholesterol, lowers blood pressure, and increases circulation.

Sally's Story

I've always loved to walk, ever since I was a young child walking to school with my friends Cathy and Nancy. In the summer, we walked to the park for swimming.

When my family moved to a Philadelphia suburb in my freshman year of high school, I walked around the neighborhood to get acquainted with my new home.

In the mid 1970s, I moved to the Lehigh Valley, Pennsylvania. After each subsequent move—to Easton, then to Bethlehem, then to Allentown—I explored my new neighborhood by walking all over.

When I moved to Bethlehem, I added a dog as my walking partner. That was more than 45 years ago, and I still walk with a furry partner. On weekdays, we walk two to three miles, and weekends, we usually walk five miles. I love being outdoors, observing nature, and exploring neighborhoods.

* Exercise even supports better digestion.

* Exercise may help you live longer!

Whew! So why aren't you exercising?

Types of Exercise

With all these benefits, how much time should be dedicated to exercising? The minimum recommended by most authorities, including the American College of Sports Medicine, is 150 minutes per week—equivalent to five 30-minute walks.[5] Of course, the more variety that you can add to your exercise routine, the better off you will be.

Walking

Walking is a great way to begin an exercise routine. It's easy: You can start out with small distances and expand. It's free: You don't need a membership to do it. And, it gets you outdoors, and hopefully with a touch of nature, which has additional benefits.

Here are some of the benefits of walking:

* Burns calories: The amount burned depends on the type of exercise, time spent, and your body weight.

* Strengthens your heart: 30 minutes a day can reduce your risk of cardiovascular disease.

* Decreases blood sugar: A short 15-minute walk after each meal is more effective than a 1¾-hour walk pre-meal.

* Eases joint pain: Exercise stimulates the lubrication of joints.

* Boosts immune function: 30 minutes of exercise per day can reduce your risk of colds and flu.

* Boosts energy: Exercise increases oxygen flow as well as hormones that help elevate energy: cortisol, epinephrine, and neo-epinephrine.

* Improve mood: Exercise can reduce anxiety, depression, and negativity.

* Increases creative thinking: It clears your head.[6]

* Improves sleep

* Increases longevity![7]

Sally's Story

Have you heard about the Law of Entropy? It is the 2nd Law of Thermal Dynamics.

As we age, our bodies lose efficiency, and we acquire more entropy. To counter this inefficiency, we need to put energy into it. Energy makes our systems more efficient. This process is considered to be negative entropy. Our ability to create physically and mentally increases our negative entropy. Therefore, it's in our best interest to continue to learn and play throughout our lives. Keep in mind that the less you use something, the less energy required, and then it becomes less used, and less efficient. The more you sit, the more likely you are to move less, moving less means less stamina, less efficient body systems, and pretty soon you're out of shape![8]

When I feel tired during the day and a nap is appealing, I instead go outside and take a walk. The walk energizes me, and the rest of my day is more productive.

Top Exercise Tips

* Wear sturdy, comfortable shoes.

* Choose loose comfortable clothing.

* If you're exercising outside in winter, check the temperature and make sure to layer up—especially your hands, face, and head.

* Carry plenty of tissues in the winter!

* If it's dark outside, wear reflective clothing or a construction yellow or green vest with reflective tape. Carry a flashlight.

* Walking trails or sidewalks is best. However, if on a roadway, make sure there is a shoulder to move to when facing oncoming traffic. Don't wear headphones. Be alert to approaching traffic. And listen to nature.

* Hydrate: Drink water prior and after exercise, even in the winter.

* Lather up with sunscreen and lip balm, regardless of the weather.

* Breathe in the fresh air and let your head clear.

* Exercising with a friend or group may result in up to 20 percent more exercise for your body. Friends help the time pass more quickly, you have more fun, challenge each other, and make a stronger commitment to exercise

* Although our bodies are designed to work best when moving, when we have a rigorous workout routine, we need to build in rest periods to allow the body to recover and rebuild.

* Make sure to vary your workouts: Some days, focus on aerobic exercise, such as walking, spinning, running, hiking, kickboxing, and cardio machines. Other days, do anaerobic exercise, such as weight training, isometrics, and high intensity interval training.

Consequences of Lack of Exercise

We were designed to move. A lack of movement gums up our internal systems.

* Blood doesn't circulate well.

* You don't get enough oxygen.

* Your digestive system gets sluggish.

Your Turn

How much exercise do you get each week? Log your exercise for a week to find out. How can you improve?

Sunday

TYPE OF EXERCISE: _____ MINUTES EXERCISED: _____

OBSERVATIONS/THOUGHTS: _____

_____

Monday

TYPE OF EXERCISE: _____ MINUTES EXERCISED: _____

OBSERVATIONS/THOUGHTS: _____

_____

Tuesday

TYPE OF EXERCISE: _____ MINUTES EXERCISED: _____

OBSERVATIONS/THOUGHTS: _____

_____

Wednesday

TYPE OF EXERCISE: _____ MINUTES EXERCISED: _____

OBSERVATIONS/THOUGHTS: _____

_____

Thursday

TYPE OF EXERCISE: _____ MINUTES EXERCISED: _____

OBSERVATIONS/THOUGHTS: _____

_____

Friday

TYPE OF EXERCISE: _____ MINUTES EXERCISED: _____

OBSERVATIONS/THOUGHTS: _____

_____

Saturday

TYPE OF EXERCISE: _____ MINUTES EXERCISED: _____

OBSERVATIONS/THOUGHTS: _____

_____

- Lymph system doesn't flow: Your lymphatic system's major "engine" is your muscle movement. The lymph system is your body's primary defense (immune) system. You don't want a stagnant immune support. When you walk, your legs become the natural pump that helps move the lymph fluid through your body.[9]
- Toxins don't get excreted. Do you need more reasons?
- Greater risk of developing high blood pressure
- Increased type 2 diabetes risk
- Feelings of anxiety and depression

Sally's Story

I don't want to rely on technology or other people to help my mobility as I age. I think of those commercials for the life alert systems. Who wants that? I want to depend on my own physical ability to not fall or be able to get up if on the floor.

How can you incorporate more moving into each day? After years of trying a multitude of options—before work, during work, before dinner, after dinner—I finally found my best routine, and I do my best to make these workouts a priority. However, sometimes life and commitments and an occasional cold will prevent me from completing this weekly routine. I've learned that just because I miss a session or two, sometimes three, doesn't mean that my routine is busted. It just means that I'm giving myself a holiday by breaking my routine, and it can make me stronger because I choose to resume it.[16]

It took me awhile to find the exercise routine that worked best for me mentally and physically. For the past 12 years, I've been pretty faithful, weight training for strength and bone density two or three mornings a week, kickboxing for cardiovascular support and balance two evenings a week, and most recently, I added yoga one evening a week for flexibility.

This last addition was a long time coming. I didn't understand the physical exertion needed for yoga. It always seemed to me to be less physical (me, who played team sports all through high school and college). However, I felt my body desiring more flexibility especially as I embrace this next chapter, or should I say, next decade of my life.

Foods for Fitness

Here are some helpful foods to support your exercise routine.

Pre-workout:

* Oatmeal and berries
* Apples and walnuts or peanut butter (preferably organic because regular can have added oils and sugars)
* Greek yogurt
* Bananas
* Protein/fruit smoothies
* Scrambled eggs

Post-workout

* Multigrain bread with peanut butter
* Honey (Yes, just straight eaten with a spoon!)
* Oatmeal
* Greek yogurt
* Quinoa with blackberries
* Pecans
* Grilled chicken
* Tuna
* Roasted vegetables
* Cottage cheese[13]

I was introduced to two excellent recipe books created by two runners: *Run Fast, Cook Fast, Eat Slow* and *Run Fast, Eat Slow*.[14] The authors published two cookbooks, and both are excellent for both pre- and post-workouts. What I like the most is that they incorporate common foods and spices. Other cookbooks I've read require minimum amounts of obscure foods/spices. Every recipe that I have made has been put through the rigorous test of appealing to my husband. So far, we are at 90 percent success rate, which I find truly amazing!

Here are some foods to avoid eating after a workout.

* Oily/high fat foods
* Red meat
* Coffee
* Sugary drinks[15]

* Risk of certain cancers:[10] Some of the dreaded illnesses of our time, cancer and chronic disease, seem to be offset through exercise. Exercise can help lower your risk of breast, colorectal, and uterine cancers by maintaining a healthy weight, regulating hormones and speeding digestion.[11]

Sally's Story

Although the focus of this section has been on walking, we should include other important exercises in our weekly routine. Walking is available to most individuals and doesn't require an investment in equipment or a gym. However, if you can (and with approval of your doctor) consider adding some additional exercises to balance your regimen.

Walking

Minimal aerobic: This is when I walk my Yorkshire Terrier, Zoey. It gets me out in the fresh air but at a snail's pace. This pace helps me to clear my head and observe nature around me. It isn't really exercise for me; it's more for Zoey.

Moderate aerobic: This is when I walk my mixed lab, Jill. We walk fast, and my breathing and heart rate are increased. This is especially true on walking up hills. I find that my ability to sing or talk is interrupted by trying to breathe! Other exercise forms that can create this level of intensity are walking on a treadmill, bike riding, dancing, or easy jogging.

How often? 5 days a week, 30 minutes per day is the most recommended regimen.

Vigorous aerobic: The pace of this means you are unable to carry on a conversation with your walking partner, at least not in full sentences, regardless of topography! You will most likely break into a sweat at some point. This is considered brisk walking and can also be obtained through jogging and biking. Since I can't run any more (torn meniscus), it is a periodic fast pace within my walk.

How often? 3 times a week for a total of 75 minutes is recommended. 150 minutes at this level would be terrific.

Strength Training

Starting in our thirties, we begin to experience "age-related" muscle mass loss. There can be illnesses associated with muscle loss, but that is not addressed here. You can build strength and muscle mass at almost any age (very important over 60), as long as you have the right routine.

Regular exercise has been found to address these chronic diseases such as heart, diabetes, asthma, back/joint pain by managing symptoms and improving health. However, prior to starting an exercise program if you have a chronic illness, check with your physician about type, level of intensity, and length.[12]

My workout includes three days of strength training per week for about 30-45 minutes each day; it is recommended that you include at least two days. I prefer to use the gym equipment, but I also have some home equipment (free weights, rubber bands, mat) in the event I can't get to the gym.

Types of strength routines: A variety including lifting, pushing, and pulling. Generally 8 to 10 different exercises with repetitions of 12 to 15 per exercise.

Initially, you may want to hire a trainer to help you develop your routine and instruct you on the proper positioning and weight use. Over time you will need to increase the amount of weight/resistance in your routine.

Flexibility and Balance

This is where I added yoga because stretching and balance had not been a part of my weekly routine. This can be done online or in person. I prefer the in-person, small group experience so that I get the positions correct.

Stretching: It is recommended that it be done at least twice a week. Included in this would be major muscle and tendon groups. Personally, I alternate this with my strength training days.

Balance: When you "forward" walk, you are engaging balance. However, after age 60, it is important to include other balance activity types such as backward or sideway walking, standing on one leg then the other (this can be done when brushing your teeth, waiting in line), or standing from a seated position. The yoga tree position is a good one. See how long you can hold it steady; I am still working on 25 seconds with a goal of 60 seconds, without wiggling to stay on one foot. And, do it barefoot. Sneakers can provide a false sense of being able to balance.

For additional age-related exercise recommendations, you can go to https://health.gov/our-work/physical-activity/current-guidelines.

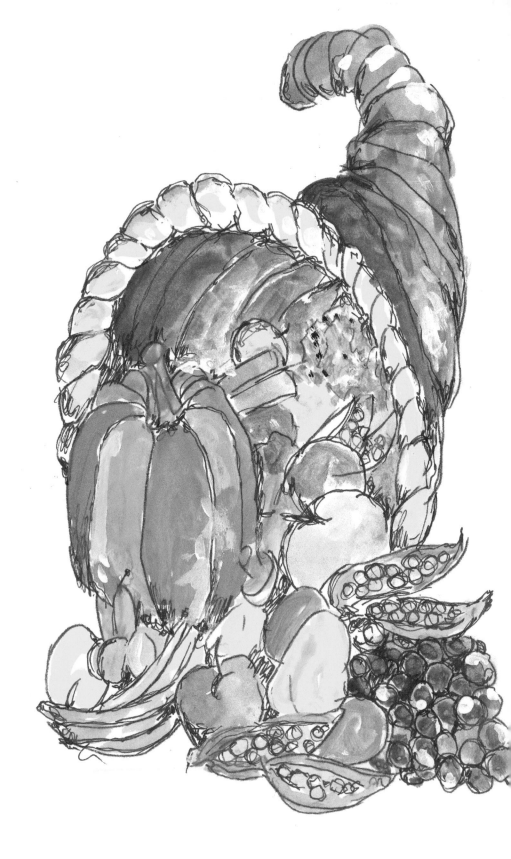

CHAPTER 4

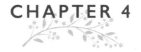

Eat

"Let food be your medicine

and let medicine be your food."

—*Quote credited to Hippocrates, 2500 years ago*

FOR MOST OF MY ADULT LIFE, I've loved food. In the past, I would have said that I live to eat, but today, it's the opposite. I eat to live. I have more knowledge now regarding food choices and their impacts on my health. And my goal is excellent health.

It's becoming more known that we are what we eat. Our bodies are great adapters. However, that doesn't mean that it's healthy adapting to a poor diet.

If you survey everyone that you know, I bet that at least 90 percent would support these common body/health goals/desires:

* Burn off stored fat
* Build and preserve muscle
* Increase energy
* Improve strength/power
* Stay well; don't get sick

If we all have similar desires, why does it seem so difficult to do?

The quality of the food that you eat can change everything! Food choices over time will affect your behavior and even the genetics of your children and grandchildren. The food that you eat will become your blood, tissue, cells, thoughts, and feelings. Your body is self-renewing.

The Importance of Good Nutrition

Over an average lifetime, we'll have eaten 25 tons of food. Our choice of food will influence our level of health and wellness. Toxins and chemicals can accumulate in our body. Our cells don't recognize them and are not sure what to do with them. Hence, these non-food elements get stored in all the wrong places until the liver can process them. Those storage areas are our fat cells (adipose tissue located between muscles and around internal organs), particularly in the abdominal cavity.[1]

Consequences of Bad Nutrition

If the quality of your food/nutritional value is lacking, you're putting your health at risk.

Most autoimmune diseases develop over extended periods of time. They slowly and gradually build up through the accumulation of "foods" the body doesn't recognize, which can get stored or reacted adversely to.

Poor nutrition lessens the body's ability to function. It can contribute to

DID YOU KNOW

Each cell in your body is replaced every seven years.[2] Seven years from now, you will be an entirely new you! Our body systems use what we eat and drink to build our blood, reinforce our cell walls. Our blood if "clean" helps with efficient use of O2 and CO2 elimination, clear thoughts, and nutrients to power our cell's mitochrondria.

What is quality food? It's food that is:

* Whole and clean, which closely resembles its natural state.

* Organic, grown without chemicals, which can be expensive, but there are ways to clean up your food choices without going totally organic.

* In season, which encourages variety as well as the season's nutritional needs. Fruits and vegetables that are in season in your area are a great choice on which to base your meal planning.

stress, tiredness, and capacity to work. Over time, unhealthy eating can contribute to the risk of developing illnesses and health problems, such as overweight or obesity, tooth decay, and high blood pressure.[3] Poor nutrition in childhood can lead to osteoporosis and cardiovascular diseases.

Types of Foods

Let's take a closer look the varying choices you have in nutrition.

Whole Foods

Choose more of these. This is defined as closest to the original source and grown or raised without chemicals, including:

* Pasture/grass fed animals: The fields in which the produce is grown or livestock has roamed should be providing the nutritional value that our bodies need.
* Whole dairy products (milk, butter, cheese, yogurt)—with no chemical processing to reduce fat content
* Wild caught (not farm-raised) fish and shellfish
* Fruit and vegetables
* Nuts
* Whole grains

Processed Foods

Avoid these. To process foods, chemicals have been added for shelf life, color, and flavoring. They are created using an "assembly line" mentality for producing the end product. Generally, the nutritional value is limited. Sometimes vitamins are added back. However, the question to consider is in what form is the added vitamin? Is it another chemical?

Sally's Story

For years, I tried a variety of diet plans. In college, I ate whatever I wanted in the cafeteria—until I went from 130 pounds to 170—and that was while being a PhysEd major and playing two intercollegiate sports.

On summer vacations, I started an early weight watching effort with an emphasis on tuna and cottage cheese. Then, while on diet pills it was toast with cheese and Fresca, which kept me very active! In my late twenties, I would periodically do the diet yo-yo. Of course, smoking helped to keep my weight down. There's nothing like a cigarette and coffee for lunch.

By the time I was 40, after quitting smoking, I knew that I needed to change my food choices. However, the choices I made didn't help: I switched to eating low-fat, low-carb foods. By age 50, I really scaled back on intake and increased my activity. That lasted for just a few months, like most of my good intentions.

At age 58, I made a conscious decision to make exercise a priority in each day. That helped with muscle tone, and I dropped a size or two. But I still hated to get on the scale—especially at the doctor's office.

By the time I was age 67, I figured that this was it. I got rid of some of my skinny wardrobe, went to some larger sizes, and tried to hide my excess weight with my clothing. A friend and trainer told me it was my food choices that were the problem, because I was exercising consistently. However, he didn't offer me any diet suggestions.

At age 68, I decided to learn more about nutrition and started the Institute for Integrative Nutrition (IIN) program, and my weight started to change. I reduced processed foods in my diet. I cooked more at home. I looked for whole, seasonal foods. In a few months, even my "barely fit" clothes were too big. I couldn't even alter them.

Today, more than a year later, my weight has been consistent to what it was after college. I still do the same exercise program that I've done for many years, but I changed my food choices. I feel better and am now discarding my "fat wardrobe." I know that I'll never wear it again!

Organic Foods

Organic foods, by definition, have been grown without chemicals, including pesticides and antibiotics. They're often in a special aisle at the store, and they're easily identified by the "Organic" label.

Organic foods are almost always more expensive than conventionally grown foods. Eat as many organic foods as you can afford.

Non-Organic Foods

As much as your budget will allow, avoid these, especially non-organic meat. When eating non-organic meat, for example, you're eating second-hand chemicals. These animals have ingested chemicals and/or antibiotics either through their food or drugs, which their bodies are unable to process. As with humans, these chemicals and/or antibiotics will be stored in their meat, organs, or fat. The majority—80 percent—of all antibiotics used are given to animals because they are being raised in bad conditions. If you believe in the "energy" factor related to all living things, intention becomes another issue.

Macronutrients

Although we're all individuals and our needs for certain micro and macro foods will vary, all bodies need protein, dietary fats, and complex carbo-hydrates for growth, building, and repair.

Diets that are restrictive of these macronutrients (protein, fat, and carbs) tend to disrupt our body's ability to function efficiently. There is a 90 to 97 percent recidivism rate on typical diet plans, which leads to the "diet bounce/rebound."

Remember as you plan your food choices, contemporary diets don't look to balance your body's health with weight loss. In your search to lose weight, learn to understand your body's needs/requirements and be careful to not jeopardize your health.

Protein: Protein builds and repairs tissues. In addition, protein also makes enzymes, hormones, and other body chemicals. Protein is an important building block of bones, muscles, cartilage, skin, and blood.[5]

Good protein sources include:

- Beans
- Lentils
- Quinoa
- Nuts

- Eggs
- Oats
- Cottage cheese
- Shellfish

- Chicken
- Beef
- Pork

Protein needs are higher when you're sick, aging, and exercising. However, eating too much protein can stress the kidneys.

Fat: Fat is the body's preferred fuel. Dietary fats are essential for body energy and the support of cell growth. Fats help protect your organs and keep your body warm. Fats are also involved in some hormone productions and nutrient absorption. Vitamin D needs dietary fats to be properly absorbed.[6] Healthy fats include:

- Avocados
- Dark chocolate
- Eggs
- Fatty fish, such as salmon, tuna, sardines, and trout

- Nuts
- Extra virgin olive oil
- Coconut and coconut oil
- Yogurt, whole milk

If you see "low-fat" on a label, beware. Low fat is engineered (chemical) fat. Low-fat diets have a negative effect on the fats and cholesterol in our blood.

Complex carbohydrates: Our bodies break down all carbohydrates into sugar, which becomes glucose. Glucose is what provides the energy for

What Are You Craving?

A craving is the body trying to create a balance for something it needs. Cravings could be attributed to:

- Fatigue
- Stress
- Lack of sleep

- Addictive foods, such as sugar or cheese

our bodies (ATP). Carbs with a lot of fiber—such as quinoa and oatmeal—are broken down slowly, which stabilizes our blood sugar levels, keeping your pancreas production of insulin stable.[7]

Complex carbohydrate foods provide vitamins, minerals, and fiber that are important to your good health. Most of your carbohydrates should come from complex carbohydrates (starches) and naturally occurring sugars, rather than processed or refined sugars, which do not have vitamins, minerals, and fiber. Refined sugars are often called "empty calories" because they have little to no nutritional value.[8]

Don't take this to mean you should eat a low-carb diet! When carbs disappear from our diets, our bodies get ready to hibernate. That means that metabolism starts to slow down, and body temperature, breathing, and heart rate decrease. This is not a desired state to maintain a healthy body—unless you're a bear.

Earlier, we talked about inflammation and its dangers (See page 34). The best food choices to reduce cellular inflammation are a balance of protein, carbs, and fat.

Here are some examples: nuts (almonds, walnuts, flax), fruits (apples, cherries, berries, grapes), tomatoes, whole grains (barley, wild rice, oats), beans (black beans, black-eyed peas, chickpeas), beets, carrots, peas, whole dark chocolate (70 percent).

Micronutrients

By definition, a micronutrient is a chemical element or substance required in trace amounts for the normal growth and development of living organisms.[9]

There are four groups of micronutrients: water-soluble vitamins, fat-soluble vitamins, macro minerals, and trace minerals.[10]

Although there are many micronutrients that could be covered here, I have chosen four that have universal impact and known deficiencies.

B6: This vitamin is needed for a healthy immune system, nerve function, and the prevention of certain types of anemia.

- At risk for deficiency: people with kidney disease, autoimmunity, and who drink too much alcohol
- Symptoms of deficiency: rash, scaly patches, dandruff, depression, confusion, and seizures

- Food sources: pork, poultry, fish, whole grains, broccoli, spinach, citrus fruits, avocados, bananas, legumes, nuts, almonds, and sunflower seeds

Iron: This mineral supports red blood cells and ability to carry oxygen-hemoglobin.

- At risk for deficiency: children and women of child-bearing age
- Symptoms of deficiency: fatigue, dizziness, headache, and chilly extremities
- Food sources: lean meat, poultry, shellfish, pumpkin seeds, quinoa, and spinach

Vitamin D: This fat-soluble vitamin (well, technically it's a hormone) supports bone health and immunity. Our bodies can produce Vitamin D if given sufficient sunlight. However, most adults lose the ability to efficiently create vitamin D.

- At risk for deficiency: adults living in areas of low sun seasons, and people with dark skin color
- Symptoms of deficiency: bone pain, muscle weakness, and increased infections
- Food sources: salmon, egg yolks, canned tuna, shrimp, and mushrooms[11]

Vitamin C: This vitamin is necessary for the growth, development and repair of all body tissues, and it is involved in many body functions, including formation of collagen, absorption of iron, function of the immune system, healing of wounds, and maintaining cartilage, bones, and teeth.[12]

- At risk for deficiency: smokers, alcoholics, people with poor diets or mental illness, people on dialysis
- Symptoms of deficiency: bleeding gums, frequent bruising, and slow wound healing[13]
- Food sources: oranges, apples, lemons, limes, potatoes, broccoli, and strawberries

Tips for Healthy Nutrition

There is no right way for everyone to eat. Unfortunately, we haven't accepted that basic foundation as the diet industry is a $110 billion dollar industry, and the food industry spends $90 million a day on advertising—both to convince us to try this method or food!

Our bodies are all different in what will work best or do harm. This "bio individualism" is founded in our individual histories: our parents, grandparents, and country of origin. We must focus on our own needs. Listen to your gut versus the diet marketing machine. Focus on nutritious food and not calories.

Here are some ways that you can begin to put clean eating into your food choices.

* We need to remember to eat plenty of whole foods—not processed, fat-free, low-sugar "junk."

* Watch your sodium intake. We tend to get too much salt in our normal diets, especially as we grow older, and your taste buds might not work as well as they used to, and you might reach for the salt-shaker to enhance the taste of your food. An acceptable daily level of salt is 1,500 milligrams per day. (Studies vary: 2,000 milligrams is noted by the Heart Foundation in Australia.[14])

   Salt has been branded as the single most dangerous mineral in our food supply. It can create hypertension/high blood pressure, which can result in heart attacks, strokes, kidney stones, dehydration, gastric ulcers, and electrolyte imbalance.

Sally's Story

I was at a diner shortly after I started Institute for Integrative Nutrition (IIN). An older couple across from our booth grabbed my attention. When their food arrived, before even taking a taste, the gentleman took the salt and applied generously. Then, to my wide-eyed amazement, he took the top off of the salt-shaker to get more. It was all I could do to hold myself back from visiting their table!

* Eliminate refined white carbohydrates: sugar, flour, and fructose syrup. There's no nutritional value to these foods. Because your body has no use for them, they tend to get stored. Sugar, in particular, can be addictive and can be related to mood swings. Some researchers have indicated that depending upon the person, sugar can be as addictive as cocaine. This doesn't mean that you can never taste sweets or bread again as there are alternatives, such as honey and coconut palm sugar for sweeteners and whole wheat for bread. (See "A Quick Note About Sugar" on page 23.)

* Cook at home as often as possible. When eating out, whether fast food or fine dining, the ingredients and preparation often include chemicals to keep the food fresher longer, make it an appealing color, etc. These foods are generally higher in calories than food made at home. Also, when you cook at home, you have a better knowledge of the source of the food.

  Contrary to the concern about having to spend a lot of time in the kitchen, there are ways to prepare and make food in advance. Here are some of my tips.

  - When making some foods, I double the recipe, allowing me to freeze some, such as muffins, tomato sauce, and meatballs and cutting up fresh fruits and vegetables.

  - When I roast a chicken, I will use it for several meals, such as roasted chicken, chicken salad, BBQ chicken, chicken soup.

  - I wash my fruit, celery, and carrots before putting them into the refrigerator, which allows me to just grab them when using in a meal.

  - I keep a small jar of peeled garlic cloves in the refrigerator at all times.

Sally's Story

Food shop with a plan, and never on an empty stomach! This was a lesson that my mother impressed on me. To this day, I try to make sure to either drink water or eat something before entering the grocery store!

Sally's Story

Experts often encourage us to make a weekly meal plan, which helps to develop the shopping list and hopefully, keep our expenditures in line. I've never been really good about that. However, I do look at the weekly store flyer and coupons, and I develop a list of basic ingredients that could have multiple dinner options.

My pantry is filled with healthy staples, such as spices (cinnamon, sea salt, pepper, oregano), extra virgin olive oil, coconut palm oil, molasses, maple syrup, and honey.

Also, I buy dry goods, such as vegetable pasta, quinoa, oatmeal, coconut palm sugar, beans/legumes, and whole wheat flour in bulk.

Consequently, I am able to prepare several options easily, quickly, and inexpensively at home.

- Avoid "diet foods," which have been chemically altered to reduce calories, fat, sugar, etc. As with white carbs, these chemical foods are not recognized by our bodies and therefore, are usually stored somewhere—most likely in fat.

- There is a system to grocery market shopping. For the most part stick to the perimeter of the store. Fresh, frozen, and refrigerated sections offer better selections than shelved packaged foods. Shelved foods tend

---

DID YOU KNOW

According to Neal Barnard, MD, head of the Physicians for Responsible Medicine:

- Chicken is not a health food.

- Cheese is 70 percent fat—saturated fat.

- Diabetes is not a genetic disease. Affected genes can turn around. Fat build-up stops insulin from working.[15]

to have more preservatives i.e. shelf life. You want to shop for foods that don't have chemicals/preservatives that you can't even pronounce. In fact, the fewer the ingredients in the food, the better it is for you.

An easy to remember hierarchy of food choices is:

- Fresh is best.
- Frozen is good if fresh is not available.
- Local is better. It tastes better and is fresher than food that has traveled a distance.
- Organic is much better than non-organic, especially if the food is clean, whole, and seasonal.

* Change the proportions of foods in your diet. Add more plant-based foods and reduce meat. Even a 10 percent change can be very beneficial. Consider having several meatless meals each week, or at minimum, a meatless Monday!

* As you take time to really read labels, it may take you a little longer to shop. After the first few times, you will begin to know the aisles and choices, which should make it less of a chore. I now enjoy my shopping adventures, and the time needed is the same or less than before.

* Do you despise food shopping? The online ordering from your local grocery store is an option. You can review ingredients online and not worry about the cart, cashing out, or bagging. However, you will still need to unbag at home.

* During the late spring, summer, and early fall, you may find some delicious whole food at a local farmers' market or a community share agriculture (CSA). This is a wonderful way to support the small independent farms in your area as well as to buy the freshest food possible.

Our Relationship with the Plant Kingdom

The relationship between plants and humans is extremely important. We are more dependent upon them than they are on us.

In essence, plants make all the food we eat, whether it is directly by eating the plant or indirectly by eating meat from an animal that ate plants. And, plants make their own food. In fact, plants are noted to use only about $\frac{1}{6}$ of the energy it gets from the sun to nourish itself; the rest of the energy is stored in the form of glucose until it is eaten by other animals or humans.[16]

Our bodies can tell the difference between natural and synthetic foods, chemicals, and drugs. We have receptors in our cells that work in concert with plants. An example is the human system of respiration and the plant system of photosynthesis. We are dependent on each other to live.[17]

If the particle is recognized as natural, the body knows how it works and where it can be used. If the particle is synthetic, the body is unable to determine its use and believes that there could be a purpose, so it is stored. Vitamins from foods and plants are more bio available to our bodies than synthetic or chemically produced vitamins and minerals.

Regardless of your beliefs in the theory of human development (religion or scientific), there is a close association of our evolution and a plant-based environment. We (humans and plants) all start as a single cell, which then divides, divides again, and so on, becoming organized for specific purposes (tissues) and functions (organs), which in humans become grouped together as systems, such as digestive, respiratory, and circulatory. We are all connected.

Sally's Story

I truly believe that we live in a "garden of Eden." Unfortunately, we have lost our knowledge of the garden and its healing ways. We have become so busy with our lives that we have come to believe that we can fix most ailments with a pill. Should it take longer than a few hours, we are not satisfied. We must remember that many prescription medications and over-the-counter drugs will only mask the problem by alleviating some or all symptoms or send the sickness deeper in the body. We must explore the root cause for the dis-ease and then work to find a way to bring the body back to homeostasis/balance.

The use of herbs/plants in a healing protocol focuses on the individual and not the disease. There are different herbs for different people who have different energy levels. There are three primary categories of herbs:

* *Food, which can be taken daily*
* *Medicine, which is for a specific reason and time*
* *Poison, which we should all avoid unless highly trained*

Plants used in herbal medicine include herb (annual, biennial, perennial), tree, shrub, vine, and weed. The parts used can be flower, fruit, leaf, stem/bark, and roots. The characteristics that herbalists recognize and value include:

* *sweet*
* *salty*
* *sour*
* *astringent*

* *pungent*
* *bitter*
* *bland*

The use of herbs in a healing protocol is selected to match the energy needed as well as components that can bring balance/homeostasis to the body. Therefore, there may be more than one part or even more than one herb used.

A note for the weeds: We have overlooked their virtues for a long time because they seem to crop up in places that we don't want them to be, such as flower beds, lawns, and vegetable gardens. Take a moment and just reflect on a few helpful "weeds":

* *Dandelion: Flower makes wine;, leaves make salad greens.*
* *Plantain: Mashed leaves can reduce the sting and inflammation from insects and bees.*
* *Chicory: It's used like coffee, especially in the southern United States.*
* *Plus consider chickweed, ground ivy, periwinkle, spice bush, and many more useful "weeds."*

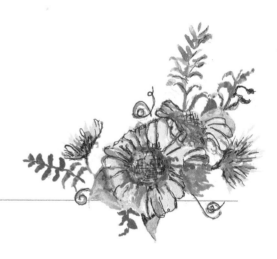

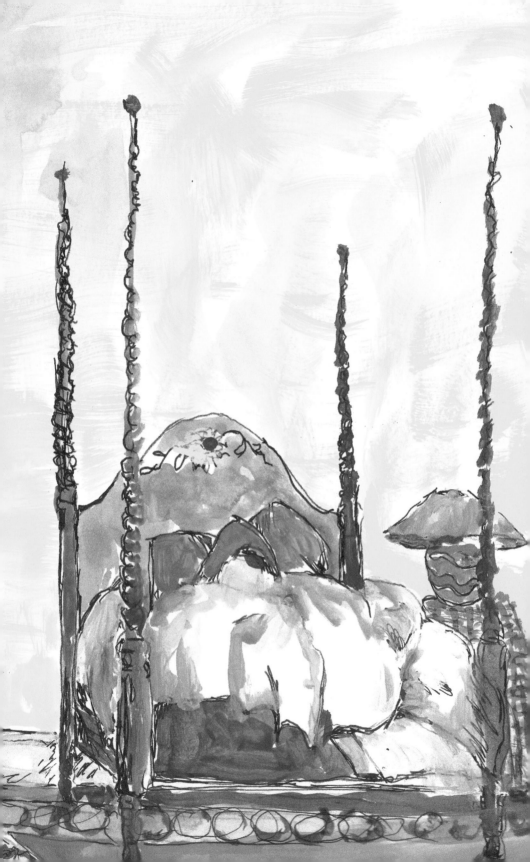

CHAPTER 5

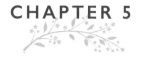

Sleep

SLEEP IS AN IMPORTANT PART of everyone's routine. We spend about one-third of our time fast asleep. Both quality and quantity of sleep are as essential to survival as food and water. Without sleep, you can't form or maintain the pathways in your brain that let you learn and create new memories. Lack of sleep makes it harder to concentrate and respond quickly.[1]

According to the Cambridge Dictionary, a succinct definition of sleep is: "the resting state in which the body is not active and the mind is unconscious."[2]

In modern times, we tend to substitute other activities for sleep—recreation, watching TV, reading, relaxing—thinking that these forms of rest help to offset sleep requirements. But they are not the same as sleep. When you're truly asleep, there is a loss of external conscientiousness and a feeling of distorted time.[3]

The Importance of Sleep

Loss of external consciousness doesn't mean your whole body is sleeping. On the contrary, sleep benefits every major organ in your body. To name a few benefits, sleep:

* Optimizes your capacity for learning
* Supports your memory
* Helps your tissues repair
* Allows for muscle growth
* Assists in protein synthesis
* Supports growth metabolism: Sleep is related to hormonal and metabolic processes.

According to Matthew Walker, PhD, a neuroscientist and professor at UC Berkley, one night of poor sleep is worse than starvation or lack of exercise.

Sleep is essential to life. In order for the body to do its maintenance, it needs at least seven to eight hours of sleep, on a consistent basis, and preferably at consistent a time of day, seven nights a week.

Circadian rhythms, which we lived by prior to the age of industrialization and electricity, helped to get humans in sync with nature. Circadian rhythm is a 24-hour rhythm that determines the sleep-wake cycle of every living organism—humans, animals, and even plants.

Yes, plants have a 24-hour circadian rhythm. Chemicals within the plant respond to sunlight and dark. At night, a plant will cease photosynthesis and continue with respiration. Night is when the glucose created during the day is distributed to other parts of the plant.

Even if you lived in total darkness, your body would have a sleep-wake cycle.

Although sleep needs are said to be hardwired into our DNA, like most things, individuals vary in their own cycles.

The World Health Organization (WHO) regards sleep loss as an epidemic in most Western nations.[4] Unfortunately, when many people have difficulty sleeping, they reach for sleeping pills. This is, at best, a short-term

Sally's Story

A critical point that I was not aware of until writing this book is that teenagers' circadian rhythms are one to three hours behind that of adults. Therefore, if teens wake at 5:30 am to get ready for school, their brains believe it to be 2:30 to 4:30 am. This doesn't allow for the full sleep cycles to be completed.

A critical point for me is getting to bed by 10 pm. If I'm up later than 10 watching TV or on a computer, I might as well pull an all-nighter because I'll have such a hard time falling asleep! I'm a morning person, and I tend to wake up around 5 am. A benefit to my early-bird ways is that it allows me to either get to the gym by 5:30 am or have a morning walk, either of which starts my day on a positive note.

Your Turn

How much sleep do you get? Keep a log for a week. Log your bedtime, time asleep, and time awoke. Note any observations, such as foods eaten or beverages drank after supper, nighttime awakenings, etc. Do you see any patterns?

Sunday

BED TIME: _____ TIME ASLEEP: _____ TIME AWAKE: _____ HOURS SLEPT: _____

OBSERVATIONS: _____

Monday

BED TIME: _____ TIME ASLEEP: _____ TIME AWAKE: _____ HOURS SLEPT: _____

OBSERVATIONS: _____

Tuesday

BED TIME: _____ TIME ASLEEP: _____ TIME AWAKE: _____ HOURS SLEPT: _____

OBSERVATIONS: _____

Wednesday

BED TIME: _____ TIME ASLEEP: _____ TIME AWAKE: _____ HOURS SLEPT: _____

OBSERVATIONS: _____

Thursday

BED TIME: _____ TIME ASLEEP: _____ TIME AWAKE: _____ HOURS SLEPT: _____

OBSERVATIONS: _____

Friday

BED TIME: _____ TIME ASLEEP: _____ TIME AWAKE: _____ HOURS SLEPT: _____

OBSERVATIONS: _____

Saturday

BED TIME: _____ TIME ASLEEP: _____ TIME AWAKE: _____ HOURS SLEPT: _____

OBSERVATIONS: _____

_____

option. This type of medication should be discussed with a physician and limited because your body can become tolerant to its use.

One out of three adults in the United States sleeps less than the recommended hours. In fact, you may know of folks who believe/boast that they are performing their best with only five hours of sleep each night. As with sleeping pills, that might work for the short-term, but the long-term impacts may lead to chronic illness.

There's a correlation between sleep, weight loss, and chronic disease. Also, junk food chemicals disrupt our sleep. Sleep and dreaming are cornerstones of health, and they are complementary and parallel to nutrition.[5]

When you think about our consumption as humans, we consume more than food. Especially today, information is a major part of our existence. Even computers require time to update, sort, and reboot. We rival computers with our brain processing power.

Phases of Sleep

No doubt over the years you have heard of the two phases of sleep. However, it's time to become reacquainted with them and their importance to your health.

NREM

Non-Rapid Eye Movement: This sleep phase dominates our early sleep period, usually from 11 pm to 3 am. During this phase, your eyes are restful, you

---

DID YOU KNOW

Although it's impossible to precisely calculate, it's postulated that the human brain consumes 100,000 words per day[6] and stores between 10 terabytes and 100 terabytes. (A terabyte is equal to about 1,000 gigabytes or about 1 million megabytes.)[7]

A healthy night's sleep benefits our brain in its "update, sort, and reboot" processing. The hippocampus has limited storage and serves as the short-term memory reserve; this needs to be offloaded daily. While the cortex, which is the recipient of the saved information, serves as the storage for our longer-term memory files.

Are You Using Your Brain?

How often have you heard that we only use 10 percent of our brains? That's an old myth, which may have been derived from some early 20th century works. Today, by using functional magnetic resonance imaging (Fmri), a person's brain activity can be measured while performing different tasks.[9]

Using this imaging technique and similar methods, researchers have shown that most of your brain is in use most of the time, even while you're performing a very simple action such as walking, and even while you're sleeping.

---

have calm/slow brain waves, and your brain storage is "scrubbed"—cleaned out of old and unnecessary neural connections.

Teenagers need more NREM to transition to adulthood. A teen's brain gets refined and matures from the back of the brain first. The frontal lobe—home to rational thinking—is the last area of the brain to develop. (No kidding!)

REM

Rapid Eye Movement occurs later in our sleep cycle, usually from 3 am to 7 am. It helps us make connections between seemingly unrelated concepts. Have you ever gone to sleep with a problem that you can't seem to address and wake up in the morning with the solution? Thank your REM sleep! This phase strengthens useful neural connections.

The quality of REM sleep affects everyone—from fetuses all the way to the elderly. Among the elderly, poor quality or quantity of this phase is often caused by medical conditions and medications.

How can you impact your sleep cycle? In addition to the circadian rhythm discussed, several chemicals and hormones impact sleep as well. We also impact our biological clock by our choices, such as travel and caffeine intake.

* Adenosine is a purine nucleoside base, most commonly recognized with the molecule adenosine triphosphate, or ATP (cell energy), and is used thoroughly throughout the entire body in general metabolism. ATP provides the energy to our cells.[10] Sleep helps to replenish energy to our bodies.

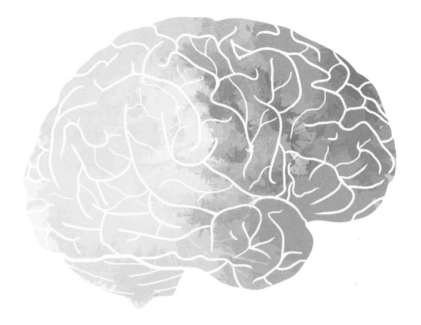

* Melatonin is a naturally occurring hormone in your body that affects your sleep-wake cycle. It's also associated with the immune system. Foods known for their melatonin content include:

  • Fruits and vegetables, such as tart cherries, corn, asparagus, tomatoes, pomegranate, olives, grapes, broccoli, and cucumber

  • Grains, such as rice, barley, and rolled oats

  • Nuts and seeds, such as walnuts, peanuts, sunflower seeds, mustard seeds, and flaxseed[11]

Over-the-counter melatonin is often mistakenly believed to help one to sleep. In essence it helps prepare the body to sleep, but it doesn't induce sleep.[12]

Consequences of Lack of Sleep

Although we may not realize it, there are some substantial impacts related to deprived sleep. Unfortunately, these may build over time so we are not as aware of their impact.

* Emotional instability: We become unable to balance positive and negative emotions.

* Bad decision making: Lack of sleep can lead to aggression, risk taking, depression, and addictions. (Is your doctor, boss, bus driver getting enough sleep?)

* Heart problems: If a person sleeps less than six hours a night consistently, research indicates that increases cardiac failure by 45 percent, increases blood pressure, and increases risk of stroke.

* Increased risk of health conditions: Lack of sleep increases risk of diabetes and weight gain, and it lowers virility and immunity.

* Loss of brain function.

* Work schedules: Shift work, early starts, and being awoken by a startling alarm can impact our heart and nervous system. For shift workers, research has found that a single night shift has cognitive effects that can last a week. A few days of reduced sleep can change your appetite, both for kinds of foods you crave and how much you want to eat when you stay awake at night.[14]

Tips for Better Sleep

According to the National Sleep Foundation, your quality of life can be enhanced with healthy sleep habits, or as they coined "good sleep hygiene."[15] The National Sleep Foundation, along with other health consultants, suggests the following to enhance the quality of our sleep.

* Develop a sleep schedule, with the same bedtime and wake up time, including weekends. This helps to regulate your body's clock and could help you fall asleep and stay asleep for the night.

* Pay attention to your sleep signals. If your body is telling you it's tired, listen and go to bed! Your sleep signals may include:[16]

  * Body position: Once you're tired, you will tend to want to become horizontal; however, some of us can begin our relaxing sitting up.

  * Reduced muscle tone: Your skeletal muscles relax.

  * Lack of overt response to external environment: You become somewhat "unconscientious."

  * Yawning: It can often be associated with fatigue.

* Have a relaxing bedtime ritual. Create a calming routine that's away from technology lights and separates sleep from other daily activities.

* Keep technology and work materials out of the bedroom. Artificial lighting and the screens from our technology (televisions, computers, cell phones) can have a REM sleep impact. The white light spectrum from these devices includes red, green, and blue. Blue light affects the melanopsin protein, which signals light is present, causing our brains to think that it is daylight; red and green do not have the same impact on this protein. Some devices now include an "evening" setting, which helps to lower or eliminate this blue light.

* Resist napping during the day because it could be impacting your night's sleep. Napping doesn't provide the full REM experience.

* Exercise. Physical exercise during the day (morning, afternoon or evening) can positively impact your sleep quality and sleep duration. It does this by reducing stress and tiring you out. Exercise is a good stress for your body.

  If performed in the morning and afternoon, exercise can help set your sleep/wake rhythm through raising your core body temperature. It's especially beneficial to your

> **DID YOU KNOW**
> Sleep deprivation is a military torture tactic?

body when you can be outside in the fresh air and sunshine. For some people, evening exercise helps to tire them out before sleep; for others it may increase their energy. Find the consistent time of day that works for your schedule and body.[17]

* Create a comfortable bedroom haven. It should be cool, quiet, and dark. However, if possible, find a way that sunlight can enter your room to provide a natural wake-up call.

* Find the best bedroom temperature. How quickly you fall asleep depends on how quickly your optimal sleep body core temperature is reached. Think about PJs, bedding, central heating; all of these can keep you from reaching your sleep core temperature. The best room temperature for sleeping is between 60°F and 67°F.

* Avoid alcohol. Alcohol suppresses REM, so if you drink, your sleep will not be continuous. Alcohol may help you to fall asleep quickly, only to waken within a few hours suppressing the REM sleep.

* Don't smoke. Nicotine is a stimulant. As such smoking can cause fragmented sleep, take longer to fall asleep, have less deep sleep, and experience more sleep disruptions.

* Don't eat heavy meals in the evening. Your digestive system needs two to three hours to work through the last meal of the day. Going to bed in less time than means that your digestive system is unable to fully repair/recover/rebuild during your sleep; it is too busy digesting that last meal.

* If you can't sleep, move to another room and do something relaxing. Sometimes a warm bath or shower might aid in getting to the sleep state.

You know the level of sleep you need and performance requirements; therefore, use your circadian schedule to your advantage.

During the "darker" time of year i.e. daylight savings in most states, during the day, get as much natural light as possible. For example, sit or work near a window and get outside when the sun is out.

* Try deep breathing. Rather than counting sheep or singing "99 Bottles of Beer on the Wall," try this breathing exercise that was recommended

by Dr. Andrew Weil and Dr. Deepak Chopra in seminars that I attended: Lie still and breathe in through your nostrils to the count of five. As you breathe in, expand your belly. Hold your breath to a count of seven. Exhale through your mouth to a count of 10. Repeat this five times. This is also is a great de-stressor anytime during the day.

* Try progressive relaxation. Concentrate on relaxing your body as you breathe deeply, hold, and exhale. Start with your toes and work your way up to the top of your head.

CONCLUSION

I **HOPE THAT IF YOU ARE READING THIS PAGE,** it's because you have read the entire book.

If so, did you notice a trend? The four major components of good health all were featured in our body systems requirements: water, exercise, quality food, and sleep. (Drink, Move, Eat, Sleep)

By changing just one of your habits, it will resonate throughout your body. It's like throwing a pebble in a pond. Imagine how your health will improve when you tackle one habit, then another, then another!

Good health isn't about a race and getting to the finish line. It's about understanding the impact of your choices. This book just scratches the surface. However, it provides a place to start by sharing an understanding of the effects and consequences of choices that you make.

Don't become a part of the CDC's statistics for 2030.* In seven years, you'll have a whole new body. Make it a good one!

If you'd like to keep in touch, please visit www.bodyconstruction.me. I post recipes and tips about organic living, wellness, and herbs. If you are so inclined, send me your experiences in these areas and become a guest blogger.

*According to the CDC, the leading cause for death in 2030 is projected to be cancer, followed by hepatitis and Alzheimer's disease. Also, projected is major depressive disorders and Ischaemic heart disease. https://www.cdc.gov/healthreport/infographics/aging/index.htm

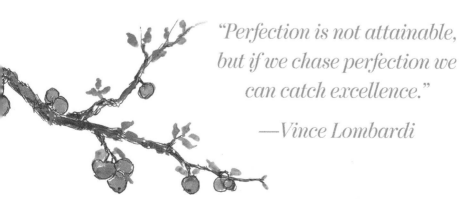

"Perfection is not attainable, but if we chase perfection we can catch excellence."

—Vince Lombardi

REFERENCES

Introduction

1. *The Promise of a New Day*, Casey, Karen, and Martha Vanceburg, Hazeden Educational Materials, 1983

2. https://www.deannaminich.com/what-to-eat-to-fuel-a-healthy-mitochondria

3. https://www.ornish.com/undo-it https://www.cdc.gov/diabetes/library/reports/reportcard.html

4. Tharp, Twyla, The *New York Times*, January 12, 2020, Living Well section, page 16

5. *Younger Next Year*, Henry S. Lodge, Workman Publishing Company, Inc., 2004

6. https://drhyman.com

Chapter 1: Body Systems

1. https://study.com/academy/lesson/what-are-the-organ-systems-of-the-human-body.html

2. https://biologydictionary.net/body-systems

3. www.drlibby.com

4. *The Body*, Bill Bryson, DoubleDay, 2019, page 95

5. *The Body*, Bill Bryson, DoubleDay, 2019, page 98

6. https://www.drfuhrman.com

7. https://rideaudental.ca/blog/education/the-four-types-of-teeth-and-their-functions-in-your-mouth.html

8. https://www.industrytap.com/stomach-acid-can-dissolve-metal/34295

9. David Winston *Herbal Therapeutics*, Herbal Therapeutics Research Library, 2003 page 34

10. http://www.biology4kids.com/files/systems_digestive.html

11. http://www.biology4kids.com/files/systems_digestive.html

12. https://www.healthline.com/health/digestion-problems#gerd

13. www.amenclinics.com

14. https://training.seer.cancer.gov/anatomy/cardiovascular

15. https://www.innerbody.com/image/cardov.html

16. http://www.biology4kids.com/files/systems_circulatory.html

17. https://www.uwhealth.org/go-red/10-ways-to-take-charge-of-your-heart-health/10543

18. https://www.dmu.edu/medterms/circulatory-system/circulatory-system-diseases

19. http://danielamenmd.com

20. http://www.bmi-calculator.net/ideal-weight-calculator/hamwi-formula

21. https://accessmedicine.mhmedical.com/content.
    aspx?bookid=575&sectionid=42512979

22. https://www.fifthsense.org.uk/psychology-and-smell

23. https://www.nursingtimes.net/clinical-archive/respiratory-clinical-archive/
    the-respiratory-system-part-1-nose-pharynx-and-larynx-23-05-2006

24. https://www.innerbody.com/anatomy/respiratory/head-neck/larynx

25. https://www.innerbody.com/image_card06/card13.html

26. https://study.com/academy/lesson/bronchi-anatomy-function-definition.html

27. https://study.com/academy/lesson/alveoli-function-definition-sacs.html

28. https://microbiologynotes.com/respiration-and-respiratory-organs

29. https://pulmonaryhypertensionnews.com/2017/12/20/8-fun-facts-lungs

30. https://www.livescience.com/22616-respiratory-system.html

31. https://www.womenhavespirit.com/article/7-ways-to-improve-respiratory-health

32. https://www.livescience.com/22616-respiratory-system.html

33. https://www.coursehero.com/file/p4lupn5/According-to-Dr-Neal-Chaisson-who-
    practices-pulmonary-medicine-at-the-Cleveland

34. *The Body*, Bill Bryson, DoubleDay, 2019 page 199

35. *The Body*, Bill Bryson, DoubleDay, 2019, page 200

36. https://www.medicalnewstoday.com/articles/303087.php

37. https://www.unitypoint.org/desmoines/article.
    aspx?id=3c97b5ba-0fe3-4616-aee1-6033a81d1c57

38. https://www.annelemonswellness.com
    blog-1/2018/2/9/2lv2hwnt0gs2im2204xc784edhvhqj

39. "The Cure for Everything," Mike Zimmerman, AARP bulletin, November
    2019, pages 112-18

40. https://www.alzheimers.net/the-stressful-life-events-that-can-lead-to-alzheimers

41. https://www.livescience.com/65342-chronic-stress-cancer.html

42. https://www.fastcompany.com/3040734/
    how-stress-shrinks-our-brains-and-what-to-do-about-it

43. https://journals.sagepub.com/doi/full/10.117⁷/0963721414535603

44. https://www.mayoclinic.org/healthy-lifestyle/stress-management/
    expert-answers/stress/faq-20058233

45. https://news.psu.edu/story/164215/2010/10/04/
    researchers-combine-knowledge-understand-stress-heart-disease

46. Joshua Rosenthal, founder, former Director, Institute for Integrative Nutrition

Chapter 2: Drink

1. https://www.everydayhealth.com/news/unusual-signs-of-dehydration
2. https://www.usgs.gov/special-topic/water-science-school/science/water-you-water-and-human-body?qt-science_center_objects=0#qt-science_center_objects
3. https://www.webmd.com/diet/features/water-for-weight-loss-diet#1
4. https://www.cnn.com/2019/03/20/health/healthiest-water-to-drink-faf/index.html
5. https://ceraproductsinc.com/blogs/the-cerasport-blog/winter-dehydration-you-can-get-dehydrated-in-cold-weather
6. www.ewg.org/tapwater
7. https://www.scientificamerican.com/article/bpa-free-plastic-containers-may-be-just-as-hazardous
8. https://www.bottledwater.org/types/bottled-water .International Bottled Water Association
9. https://www.myrecipes.com/extracrispy/whats-the-difference-between-sparkling-water-and-seltzer
10. https://www.healthline.com/nutrition/purified-vs-distilled-vs-regular-water
11. https://www.healthline.com/nutrition/purified-vs-distilled-vs-regular-water
12. https://www.tyentusa.com/blog/acidic-water-negative-effects
13. https://www.mayoclinic.org/healthy-lifestyle/nutrition-and-healthy-eating/expert-answers/caffeinated-drinks/faq-20057965
14. https://www.webmd.com/parenting/features/healthy-beverages#1
15. https://www.healthline.com/health/does-alcohol-dehydrate-you
16. https://wholefully.com/lemon-water
17. https://www.healthline.com/nutrition/19-hydrating-foods
18. https://smilesonalaska.com/2017/02/27/lemon-juice-good-bad-sour
19. https://www.cdc.gov/healthywater/drinking/nutrition/index.html
20. www.watercure.com

Other readings:

* *Back to Eden, Jethro Kloss, c1971 Benedict Lust Publications*
* *Counsels on Diet & Foods, Ellen G. White, c1938 , Ellen G White Estate Inc.*

Chapter 3: Move

1. https://www.womansday.com/health-fitness/g2318/healthy-lifestyle-quotes
2. Ncbi.nim.nih/PMC/articles/PMC1424733
3. Lexico.com/en/definition/recreation
4. *Younger Next Year,* Chris Crowley and Henry S. Lodge, M.D., Workman Publishing Company, 2004

5. http://www.acsm.org/blog-detail/acsm-blog/2017/05/16/science-of-exercise

6. https://www.healthline.com/health/benefits-of-walking

7. www.terrywalters.net

8. https://opentextbc.ca/physicstestbook2/chapter/entropy-and-the-sec-ond-law-of-thermodynamics-disorder-and-the-unavailability-of-energy

9. https://nutritiouslife.com/nurture-yourself/lymphatic-system-lose-weight

10. hopkinsmedicine.org/health/conditions-and-diseases/risks-=of-physical-inactivity

11. mdanderson.org/prevention-screening/manage-your-risk/physical-activity

12. mayoclinic.org/health-lifestyle/fitness/in-depth/exercise-and-chronic-disease/art-20046049

13. https://www.healthline.com/nutrition/eat-after-workout

14. *Run Fast, Eat Slow*, Shalane Flanagan and Elyse Kopecky, Rodale, 2016; Cook Fast. Eat Slow, Rodale, 2018

15. https://www.byrdie.com/what-to-eat-after-a-workout

16. "The Promise of a New Day," Casey, Karen and Martha Vanceburg, Hazeden Educational Materials, December 26

Chapter 4: Eat

1. https://www.huffpost.com/entry/liver-health_b_3132148
   https://www.thoughtco.com/adipose-tissue-373191] adipose

2. https://www.livescience.com/33179-does-human-body-replace-cells-seven-years.html

3. https://lwww.sahealth.sagov.au/healthyt&living

4. www.drfurhman.com

5. www.webmd.com

6. www.heart.org/healthy-living/healthy-eating/eatsmart

7. https://health.clevelandclinic.org -how carbohydrates can affect your heart

8. medlineplus.gov/envy/imagepages/192529

9. https://www.lexico.com/en/definition/micronutrient

10. https://www.healthline.com/nutrition/micronutrients

11. https://www.healthline.com/nutrition/9-foods-high-in-vitamin-d#section1

12. https://www.webmd.com/diet/features/the-benefits-of-vitamin-c

13. https://www.healthline.com/nutrition/vitamin-c-deficiency-symptoms

14. https://www.heartfoundation.org.au/healthy-eating/food-and-nutrition/salt

15. https://www.pcrm.org

16. library.thinquest.org/5420/cellsplit

17. https://www.pressconnects.com/story/news/local/2015/01/10/humans-trees-vital-relationship/21551347/

Other reading

* *The Botany of Desire, Michael Pollan, Random House 2002*

Chapter 5: Sleep

1. https://www.ninds.nih.gov/Disorders/Patient-Caregiver-Education/Understanding-Sleep

2. dictionary.cambridge.org/us/dictionary/English/sleep

3. *Why We Sleep*, Walker Matthew, PhD, Simon & Schuster, 2017

4. https://www.esquire.com/uk/life/fitness-wellbeing/a18577/sleep-loss-epidemic-insomnia-treatment

5. Joshua Rosenthal, founder past director IIN module 14

6. https://www.zdnet.com/article/americans-consume-100000-words-of-information-each-day-study-says

7. https://www.scientificamerican.com/article/what-is-the-memory-capacity

8. https://thumbnails-visually.netdna-ssl.com/major-parts-of-human-brain_53f851bd837a7_w1500.jpg

9. https://www.medicalnewstoday.com/articles/321060.php#the-10-percent-myth

10. https://www.ncbi.nlm.nih.gov › books › NBK519049

11. https://www.alaskasleep.com/blog/foods-for-sleep-list-best-worst-foods-getting-sleep

12. https://nccih.nih.gov/health/melatonin#hed2

13. "How daylight savings time can damage your health," Lindsey Tanner, *The Morning Call*, 11/3/19, page 25

14. *"Your Schedule could be Killing You,"* L. Kaufman, *Popular Science*, September/October 2017, https://popsci.com/your -schedule-could-be-killing-you

15. https://www.sleepfoundation.org/articles/healthy-sleep-tips

16. https://www.medicalnewstoday.com/articles/318414.php

17. https://www.sleep.org/articles/exercise-affects-sleep

Other reading

* *Summary and Analysis of Why We Sleep – Guide to the book by Matthew Walker*

* *The Circadian Code, Satchin Panda, PhD, 2018*

* *The Body, Bill Bryson, 2019*

* *AARP.org Bulletin November 2019, "The Cure for EVERYTHING" p11-18*

PANTRY GUIDE

Minimally processed, organic

Spices and Condiments

- ☐ Cayenne
- ☐ Cinnamon
- ☐ Garlic powder
- ☐ Ketchup, low sodium
- ☐ Mustard
- ☐ Onion powder
- ☐ Oregano

- ☐ Parsley
- ☐ Pepper
- ☐ Salt, fine sea and iodized
- ☐ Soy sauce, low sodium
- ☐ Teriyaki sauce, low sodium
- ☐ Turmeric
- ☐ Worcestershire sauce, low sodium

Refrigerator Staples

- ☐ Butter
- ☐ Carrots
- ☐ Celery*
- ☐ Eggs
- ☐ Feta
- ☐ Garlic

- ☐ Ginger
- ☐ Lemons
- ☐ Milk, whole
- ☐ Parmesan
- ☐ Onions
- ☐ Yogurt

Vegetable Staples (in season, organic, frozen)

- ☐ Apples
- ☐ Avocado
- ☐ Bananas
- ☐ Cauliflower
- ☐ Lettuce*

- ☐ Oranges
- ☐ Squash
- ☐ Tomatoes—also canned-diced, sauce, paste
- ☐ Yams/sweet potatoes

Meats/Seafood (pasture raised, organic if available)

- ☐ Chicken, dark meat
- ☐ Crab
- ☐ Beef/bison

- ☐ Fish**—wild salmon
- ☐ Shrimp

*https://www.ewg.org/foodnews/dirty-dozen.php
** www.seafoodwatch.org

Baking

- ☐ Baking soda
- ☐ Baking powder, no aluminum
- ☐ Coconut milk
- ☐ Dried fruit: apricots, dates, figs, raisins
- ☐ Flour: whole wheat (brown or white), oatmeal (cereal can be made into flour), almond
- ☐ Nuts/seeds: walnuts, almonds, peanuts
- ☐ Whole grains: quinoa, brown rice, oats
- ☐ Beans, dried: chickpeas, black, cannellini

Sweeteners (check for added sugars; get minimal)

- ☐ Black strap molasses
- ☐ Coconut palm sugar
- ☐ Maple sugar
- ☐ Honey, raw, local is best

Oils

- ☐ Avocado
- ☐ Coconut
- ☐ Extra virgin olive
- ☐ Safflower

Tips:

- ✴ Shop the perimeter of the store.
- ✴ Look for "whole" foods—not low calorie, low fat; these have chemically altered ingredients.
- ✴ Watch for added sugars; get minimal.
- ✴ If not in season (i.e. fresh), buy frozen foods.
- ✴ The fewer number of ingredients, the better.
- ✴ Remember: Your body needs carbohydrates, protein, and fat in your diet; look for the healthy and nutritional ones.

EXERCISE GUIDE

Goal: To get a daily minimum of 30 minutes of dedicated exercise* (If you have a desk job, include a goal to get up and move around every 20–40 minutes; note this isn't included in your daily 30 minutes.)

Important: Vary your workouts to allow muscle groups to recover (48 to 72 hours).

Timing: Determine the best time of the day that you can commit to a regular time of 30 to 60 minutes. Morning, afternoon and evening all have benefits; it just depends on your preferences.

Key exercise areas:

- ☐ Cardio (C)
- ☐ Balance (B)
- ☐ Strength (S)
- ☐ Flexibility (F)

Exercise benefits:

- ☐ Bicycling B.C
- ☐ Cross Fit B, C, S
- ☐ Jogging B, C
- ☐ Kickboxing B, C, S
- ☐ Roller-skating B, C
- ☐ Swimming C, F
- ☐ Tai Chi B, F, S
- ☐ Walking B, C
- ☐ Weight-lifting C, S
- ☐ Yoga B, F, S
- ☐ Zumba B, C

If you are new to dedicated exercise or have a chronic health condition, check with your physician prior to starting any exercise.

Sunday

TYPE OF EXERCISE: _____ MINUTES EXERCISED: _____

OBSERVATIONS/THOUGHTS: _____

_____

Monday

TYPE OF EXERCISE: _____ MINUTES EXERCISED: _____

OBSERVATIONS/THOUGHTS: _____

_____

Tuesday

TYPE OF EXERCISE: _____ MINUTES EXERCISED: _____

OBSERVATIONS/THOUGHTS: _____

_____

Wednesday

TYPE OF EXERCISE: _____ MINUTES EXERCISED: _____

OBSERVATIONS/THOUGHTS: _____

_____

Thursday

TYPE OF EXERCISE: _____ MINUTES EXERCISED: _____

OBSERVATIONS/THOUGHTS: _____

_____

Friday

TYPE OF EXERCISE: _____ MINUTES EXERCISED: _____

OBSERVATIONS/THOUGHTS: _____

_____

Saturday

TYPE OF EXERCISE: _____ MINUTES EXERCISED: _____

OBSERVATIONS/THOUGHTS: _____

_____

RELAXING HOME GUIDE

Natural light: Try to maximize the natural light in your living space. Depending upon weather and neighbor proximity, minimal window treatments should be considered.

Indoor lighting: Soft LED lighting is preferable to white LED at night. White light will counter the natural circadian schedule.

Technology lighting: Use a night shift option to display a warmer end of the color spectrum after dark. Limit devices in sleeping areas.

Air quality: Do you need a humidifier or de-humidifier; can you periodically open windows to allow fresh air in?

Indoor plants: Some plants that help remove chemicals from our indoors include:

- [ ] English ivy: full shade or full sun
- [ ] Bamboo palm: part shade or part sun
- [ ] Spider plant: bright or indirect light
- [ ] Mother-in-law tongue: versatile
- [ ] More examples at: hgtv.com.design/remodel/interior-remodel/10-best-plants-for-cleaning-indoor-air

Temperature: 68°F to 72°F is generally considered comfortable. Bedroom should be at the lower temperature when sleeping.

Color: Are your walls painted/papered in calming colors and prints? If painting, use a VOC-free paint.

Organized/ordered: From drawers to closets to countertops, a visual scan should reveal an uncluttered view. Spring and fall housecleaning used to be the primary force behind this effort. Consider instituting your own timing for this activity.

SAFER AND GREENER CLEANING

The following recipes are taken from EWG.org

Make your own cleaning materials:

☐ White Vinegar

☐ Baking Soda

☐ Lemon Juice

☐ Liquid soap, fragrance free and not antibacterial

☐ Washing soda*

Cleaning tools:

☐ squeegee—showers, windows, mirrors

☐ scrub brush

☐ microfiber cloth and sponge

All purpose cleaner: Mix hot water with $\frac{1}{2}$ teaspoon of washing soda and $\frac{1}{2}$ teaspoon of liquid soap or dish detergent

Bathroom: Wet $\frac{1}{2}$ cup baking soda with a small amount of liquid soap to get an "icing" consistency. Works like a soft scrub

Kitchen: Mix vinegar and salt for a grease fighting surface cleaner.

Pans: For burned on food particles in pans, sprinkle with baking soda and add about 1 teaspoon of white vinegar and let it sit.

Laundry: Instead of softener, add vinegar to rinse cycle. It prevents static cling, softens and brightens. Sprinkle dryer balls with a few drops of essential oil lavender, citrus, or thieves.

* - www.ewg.org/guides/cleaners ** - use gloves when handling washing soda

PDF copies of these forms are available on www.bodyconstruction.me.

ABOUT THE AUTHOR

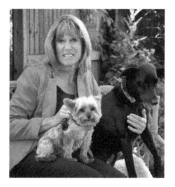

SALLY HANDLON has been an active member of the Lehigh Valley business community and non-profit community for more than 40 years. During that time, she became familiar with wellness and the environment, both of which became passionate hobbies of hers. In 2018, she made the choice to make those avocations a larger part of her life. She made her company, Handlon Business Resources (HBR), part-time and increased her focus on wellness and the environment. With that focus came the creation of www.bodyconstruction.me and her desire to write a book that would share the information she gathered over 30 years.

Sally is the founder and president of Handlon Business Resources (HBR) LLC, a WBENC certified business, located in the Lehigh Valley, Pennsylvania. HBR serves as a short-term project management partner to executives and business owners in implementing the long, overdue recommendations to move the company forward. In Stephen Covey's matrix, HBR addresses the important, non-urgent priorities. Sally started a new division in 2019 trading as Body Construction LLC.

Sally is a 2014 recipient Lehigh Valley Economic Development Corporation MVP, 2014 recipient of the YWCA of Bethlehem Woman of the Year, 2011 recipient of the Lehigh Valley Suites Award for Management Consulting, 2007 recipient of the PA Best 50 Women in Business, 2004 recipient of the US Small Business Administration Women In Business Advocate–Philadelphia Region, *The Morning Call*'s–Lehigh Valley "30 Who Shape the Valley" and "Women to Watch" as well as *Niche Magazine*'s Top 100 Retailers Nominee. Other awards include the Chamber's Athena Award (1988) and The Hillside School Service Award (1996).

Sally's civic and business activity has spanned Allentown, Bethlehem, and Easton, Pennsylvania. Her current Board activity includes: Rising Tide Community Loan Fund Board, WDIY Board and LVEDC Local Sourcing and Business Diversity Council.

Sally was active on the Lehigh Valley Economic Development Corporation's General Board for six years and chaired the Local Sourcing and Business Diversity Council for eight years. She was on the Board of the Moravian Book Shop and Women's Leadership Institute at Cedar Crest College Advisory Board. She also served on the Business Advisory Committee for the Mayor of Bethlehem. Additional board experience includes: Greater Lehigh Valley Chamber, Small Business Council, DBA- Bethlehem Merchants Association, SouthSide Film Institute, South Bethlehem Historical Society, Executive Women's Council, Allentown YWCA, Allentown Neighborhood Housing Association and The Hillside School. She has been keynote speaker at area events as well as presented position papers at the American Bankers Association in Atlanta, Retail Lending conference in Boston and the Iacocca Institute at Lehigh University. She is a past senior seminar advisor for Cedar Crest College. She is a founding member of the Women's Business Council of the Chamber (1982) as well as co-founding south Bethlehem's First Friday in 1998.

Since 2009, Sally has been a community host on WDIY 88.1 FM (NPR) for a monthly radio show that focuses on business in the Lehigh Valley, Lehigh Valley Discourse.

A graduate of Penn State University with postgraduate business courses at Muhlenberg College and Bucknell University, Sally's varied employment experience includes: financial services, call center management, retail and commercial lending, higher education, community and institutional recreation, community health planning, retail business owner, corporate mergers and acquisitions. She is a graduate of David Winston's Center for Herbal Studies, two year and graduate program. She is also one of eight in the US (18 worldwide) accredited as Excellence Audit Facilitator with the Tom Peters Future Shape of the Winners program. She is also a graduate of the Institute for Integrative Nutrition, the world's largest nutrition school and has Integrative Nutrition Health Coach certification.

ABOUT THE ARTIST

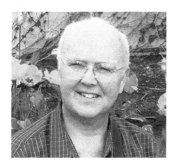

ROBERT L. HUETTER, Illustrator/Artist/Interior Designer.

I first met Bob when working for the City of Bethlehem Recreation Department in 1974. He was a summer lifeguard/pool manager and an interior design instructor in the Community Schools program. He was involved in helping to put "interior design" elements in three of my homes—and these design have remained in place and still exist today. I often tease Bob that my current home should have a placard to acknowledge that it is a "Robert Huetter original" inside and out, similar to Frank Lloyd Wright's homes.

In late 1990s, when the concept of Legends, Traditions and Friends, a gift gallery celebrating local talent and spirit, was developing, Bob worked alongside me to make it a reality. After it opened, Bob often helped in the gallery when I needed a break.

When this book started to become a reality, I knew that the illustrations had to be from Bob. He has known me a long time and understands my direction.

When I asked Bob for his bio to include with this book, he gave me a very concise description:

Robert L Huetter
Illustrator/Artist
Born in Green Bay, Wisconsin
Studied fine art at the University of Wisconsin, University of Miami, Florida and Florida Atlantic University Classical art at the Barnstone Studios in Coplay, PA Interior Designer/Owner of Panache Custom Interiors.

In keeping with the energy of *Your Journey to Aging Well*, I had to provide you, my reader, with some insight as to the illustrator.

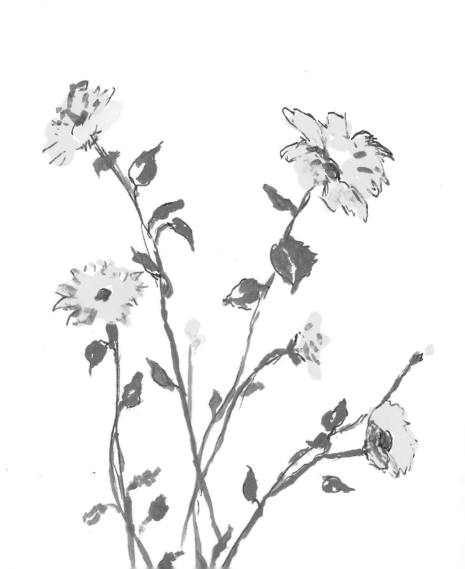

PRAISE FOR
YOUR JOURNEY TO AGING WELL

I finished Sally's book last night. Thank you for letting me get the preview. It is everything you have been telling—all wrapped up in a nice package. I can't wait to see the final print and celebrate with Sally. Congratulations on being a wonderful author.

—DANIELLE

I wasn't sure what to expect when Sally said she was writing about nutrition and health. As a person who sees myself as somewhat healthy, Sally's book definitely brought to light a few of my missing pieces. I never thought of "healthy" as a connect-the-dots to success. I am looking forward to completing the puzzle and feeling better-aging well.

—ROBIN

Sally did such a great job of organizing all this information in an enjoyable read that I think most people, who are somewhat knowledgeable about health, can enjoy. I think it is presented so clearly that even those who are new to health-related topics will be able to recognized their weak areas and follow your suggestions. There was so much information in this, but it's easy to access because Sally divided the material into the four main topics. Most importantly, there is not one tiny bit of preaching here, so everyone will be open to the information presented, and they should be grateful for Sally's expertise and sharing of her knowledge. I really enjoyed the "Sally Stories," which humanized the material.

—CATHY

It is abundantly clear that the US population is suffering from a myriad of illnesses: obesity, diabetes, heart failures, cancer, and the list goes on. What is a person to do? As we mature into the senior segment of our lives, our past lifestyle choices seem to compound and not often in the way we like! There is a wealth of publicized diet plans, "healthy" home delivered meals, and products touting low calorie counts or low sodium and health benefits through additives. All of these are "tried and true"; just listen to your favorite actor telling you the benefits of their solution. Add to that list the impact of pesticides, genetically modified foods, organic foods, and step counters. And how about all that sugar in sodas, health drinks, desserts, etc.? Then of course the number of gyms, personal trainers, exercise equipment, and exercise regimes is constantly increasing. It is overwhelming and makes one tired just thinking about it. Our lives are busier than ever. How does one fit a healthy lifestyle into their schedule?

The answer is not as complicated as you may think. You don't have to bury yourself in a book of physiology, followed by a course in nutrition, and then try out the many exercise options. Your Journey to Aging Well, authored by Sally Handlon, simplifies both the physiology of our bodies and how to best migrate to (not JUMP into) a program focusing on a healthy living lifestyle. Based on Ms. Handlon's personal health journey, her research into how our intricate bodies operate, her study of the impact of long-used herbs, and her study of nutrition and exercise, she provides a primer into modifying life choices to direct you to healthy living. This is not a "do as I say" sermon. It is a commentary of her personal experiences in finding and adopting a way to make healthy choices.

Join Ms. Handlon on a review of her journey, the trials and tribulations of getting to a place of renewed energy, maintenance of a healthy weight and a sense of wellbeing, aided by knowing you are providing your human engine with the right fuel.

—CONNIE

CPSIA information can be obtained
at www.ICGtesting.com
Printed in the USA
BVHW020156030620
580831BV00018B/920